NATURAL SOLUTIONS TO MENOPAUSE

How to stay healthy before, during and beyond the menopause

MARILYN GLENVILLE
PhD

RODALE

This edition first published 2011 by Rodale
an imprint of Pan Macmillan, a division of Macmillan Publishers Limited
Pan Macmillan, 20 New Wharf Road, London N1 9RR
Basingstoke and Oxford
Associated companies throughout the world
www.panmacmillan.com

ISBN 978-1-905744-68-8

1 3 5 7 9 8 6 4 2

A CIP catalogue record for this book is available from the British Library.

Text designed and set by seagulls.net

Printed and bound in Great Britain by CPI Mackays, Chatham ME5 8TD

This book is intended as a reference volume only, not as a medical manual.
The information given here is designed to help you make informed decisions about
your health. It is not intended as a substitute for any treatment that you may have
been prescribed by your doctor. If you suspect you have a medical problem,
we urge you to seek competent medical help.

Mention of specific companies, organisations or authorities in this book does not
imply endorsement of the publisher, nor does mention of specific companies,
organisations or authorities in the book imply that they endorse the book.

Addresses, websites and telephone numbers given in this book
were correct at the time of going to press.

Visit **www.panmacmillan.com** to read more about all our books and to buy them.
You will also find features, author interviews and news of any author events, and you can
sign up for e-newsletters so that you're always first to hear about our new releases.

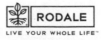

We inspire and enable people to improve their lives and the world around them

PRAISE FOR MARILYN GLENVILLE

'[You are] a wonderful breath of fresh air in the confusing world of the menopause and HRT. I have acted upon, and benefited immensely from your advice – thank you.'

'There are so many factors that affect our health and sometimes it is mind-boggling trying to figure out what is the best treatment. It is reassuring to know that Dr Glenville advises us on the issues that affect women in a simplified, interesting and informative way.'

'Excellent information available from Marilyn Glenville. I have several of her books and have found them most helpful.'

'I just want to say "thank you" for the information. So many times I have asked my doctor for info and she has just seemed to want to give me a pill or take something out! I wish I had found your website before I had a total hysterectomy five years ago. I am just glad I found it now. I stopped HRT three months ago after seven years of it. Thanks again so very much.'

'I love your writing – so simple and clear, unpatronising and really relevant. It's really helped me to help my family stay on track health-wise.'

'My main health problem to date has been the menopause – however I was fortunate to attend a seminar given by Marilyn Glenville at just the right time and the advice and information offered there and subsequently in her books got me through. I realised when talking to my own GP that this information is not out there for everybody and still wonder what my outcome might have been.'

'I have been aware of Marilyn Glenville's work for ten years now and indeed have been treated by her on several occasions. I find her a very sane, sensible and interesting practitioner and I trust in her judgement . . . the issue that interests us all is how to age well and healthily and that prevention is far better than cure.'

To my grandson Jack (born February 2010)

The joy of a new life

With love from Nana

CONTENTS

WHY THE BUTTERFLY?

The butterfly is a powerful symbol of change and new beginnings. I chose to include it in this book to reflect my vision of the menopause: a natural transition that moves you into a new stage of your life. Change is inevitable for us all, but by making the right choices it can be a time to flourish and celebrate being a woman in the best of health.

ACKNOWLEDGEMENTS

I wrote this book because, at 58 and having gone through the menopause, I felt that nothing much had been written on helping women with the next stage in their lives. It was almost as if that was it – got the T-shirt, game over. But of course we're living longer than ever and this book has been written to help women go on to enjoy a healthy and energetic future.

Nutritional medicine is such an exciting science; it's growing and developing continually, so it's vital to stay open and flexible to new ideas. New research may completely contradict theories that have been accepted as 'the truth' for years. For example, 'fat causes heart disease (and makes you overweight)' is a theory that we have to reconsider (I will look at it in detail later in the book), but changing an entrenched concept can be as slow as turning an ocean liner.

Nowhere is this better illustrated than the story of the two scientists who discovered that it was the *Helicobacter pylori* bacterium that caused stomach ulcers and *not* excess acid caused by stress or spicy foods. It took them nearly 25 years to get this concept accepted by the medical profession, as the established thinking was that no bacteria could survive in the stomach because the acid was so strong. In frustration, one of the scientists finally had to swallow a culture of *H. pylori* to prove that the bacteria could survive under those conditions!

So, as I list all the people to whom I owe my thanks, my gratitude and appreciation goes to all those scientists and researchers who, despite facing criticism and doubt from their peers, are still brave enough to raise their heads above the parapet, and risk having them knocked off.

It has been a pleasure working with my new publishers, Macmillan, and especially with my two editors, Liz Gough (who went off to have a baby) and Cindy Chan who took over seamlessly from her.

I would especially like to thank my team of nutritionists (Alison Belcourt, Helen Heap, Sharon Pitt and Lisa Smith) who work in the London and Tunbridge Wells clinics and who take such good care of the patients. Also to all the staff in Tunbridge Wells, including Wendy, Brenda, Alex, Gayla, Marian, Shirley, Lucy, Lee, Sophia and Maggie, who work so efficiently behind the scenes. Thanks also to the nutritionists in Ireland, Heather Leeson and Sally Milne, who are doing a wonderful job of looking after the women over there.

Thanks go especially to all of my patients, who have taught me so much over the years. During that time we've become very close and although nowadays I only see some of them once a year for a nutritional MOT, their impact on my life and work has been of incalculable importance. Their ability to talk about very intimate problems with a sense of humour has earned my enduring respect. I especially want to thank those women who have kept me on my toes, not only in the clinic but also at talks, by asking searching questions. They don't just accept what they are told. They want to know why! They want to understand what is going on in their bodies and to use the information to make informed decisions about their health.

Last but not least, my love goes to my family: Kriss, my husband, and my three children Matt (and his wife Hannah and their children Katie and Jack), Len and Chantell.

'Discovery consists of seeing what
everybody has seen and thinking
what nobody has thought'

Albert Szent-Györgyi, 1937 Nobel Laureate
in Physiology and Medicine

INTRODUCTION

I have written books on many different aspects of women's health and with this one I wanted to help every woman from around the age of 40, no matter which stage of the menopause she is at: whether she is approaching it, going through it or experiencing life beyond the menopause. My aim is to help you manage each stage of this natural process and to be in the best health you can be at all times, able to effectively manage any symptoms that might occur as you progress through the phases of the menopause.

My natural solutions for this chapter of life are particularly relevant if you bear in mind that we can now live anywhere between 30 and 50 years after the menopause; it is important to be able to spend these years enjoying a good quality of life with, perhaps most crucially, good health. This means living free from disease and having the energy to do the things you want to do, being free from aches and pains, having good skin and hair, sleeping well, not feeling depressed, avoiding osteoporosis, enjoying a good sex life and being on the ball mentally in terms of memory and concentration.

I see women of all ages in my clinic, and it is clear that the earlier you start to look after yourself, and are able to anticipate the changes ahead, the easier the menopause transition will be and the better your health will be *after* the menopause. It is my firm belief that using natural ways to help you manage this change is the key to good health both now and in the future – to help prevent problems in the short- and the long-term. My expertise lies in the area of nutritional medicine, and my aim is to help you enjoy a smooth menopause journey, no matter which stage of the menopause you are at.

THE MENOPAUSE JOURNEY

This book is aimed at all women from around the age of 40. It will take you right through the stages of the menopause, from before the menopause, through the changes that occur during the menopause and then beyond. It does not matter where you are in the journey when you pick up this book. My aim is to give you the tools to help alleviate menopausal symptoms and also to work on preventing health problems; the idea is that you can just turn straight to the part of the book that applies to you for guidance. By referring to the other parts of the book, you may find explanations for why you have been feeling a certain way, or you may find it helpful to read ahead to prepare for the next stage so that you can feel in control about the changes that are happening in your body.

Although I have given approximate timings for each different stage of the menopause, in reality this can only be a guide because some women will go through the stages earlier while others will experience them later, and that is completely normal. The symptoms you are experiencing will indicate the stage you are in. The only exception to this is for those women who go through a premature menopause (usually referred to as premature ovarian failure), which occurs in 1 to 4 per cent of women under the age of 40. I have included a separate section for women who have gone through an early menopause (see page 115).

You may associate going through the menopause and beyond as becoming 'old' and linked to poor health; and you may think that you will begin to age very quickly. This is not necessarily the case. Of course, as we get older, more things can go wrong with our health, but it is not inevitable that we will have poor health. The menopause is a natural stage of change in every woman's life, not a stage of decline.

No matter what age you are now, think of yourself at a crossroads: one path is the path to good health – it requires you to take responsibility for your health but the benefits are enormous. The other path is the one to degenerative diseases such as heart disease, cancer, osteoporosis, arthritis, Alzheimer's and diabetes. I have added arthritis to this list because although it is common this does not mean to say that it has to be normal or inevitable. You need to make a conscious choice either to take steps to good health or leave yourself open to the diseases listed above. If you have already had a previous episode of cancer, for example, you need to aim to prevent a recurrence and if you are Type 2 diabetic then you need to focus your efforts on keeping yourself as healthy as possible.

Remember, people rarely die of 'old age' in the West, but tend to die of illnesses that have taken time to develop over a number of years. For example, we know from research from the World Cancer Research Fund in 2009 that 80,000 people worldwide diagnosed with cancer each year could have avoided the disease by changing their lifestyle – 39 per cent of the 12 major cancers are preventable through better nutrition and lifestyle habits (that includes 19,000 cases of breast cancer and 16,000 of bowel cancer). Changes to your diet, your lifestyle and your habits really can make a difference and mean real and lasting improvements to your health.

CASE STUDY: SALLY'S STORY

'My periods stopped quite abruptly at the age of 48 and I was suddenly faced with hot flushes and night sweats. I visited my doctor because the night sweats were stopping me from sleeping, which was really affecting my energy and mood. She ran some routine blood tests and told me I was going through the menopause. I was quite shocked, as I thought the menopause was a gradual transition and that my periods would gradually wind down. She explained that with some women their periods just stop and with others the cycle becomes more irregular and then stops.

'My doctor talked to me about HRT but I knew that this was something I never wanted to take – no matter how bad my symptoms were. I was prone to lumpy breasts (fortunately just benign), but had heard that HRT could make this worse. However, I knew I had to do something to help myself because the symptoms were impacting on my daily life.

'I searched "Natural Menopause" on the internet and it led me to Dr Marilyn Glenville's website where I downloaded some very useful information. It all made so much sense and I began to feel really positive in that I was actually embarking on a new chapter in my life rather than seeing it as the end of being a woman. This really inspired me.

'I then booked an appointment at Dr Glenville's clinic. My diet was given a lot of attention and her first observation was about my intake of caffeine and alcohol – both of which are known to worsen hot flushes and night sweats as they widen the blood vessels and bring more blood to the surface of the skin producing reddening. I really loved my cups of coffee and glass of red wine, but I knew I had to make some compromises in order to feel well.

'The second area she looked at was my blood sugar. It was noted that I was eating very little protein in my diet and I was often skipping meals. She explained that something as basic as blood sugar imbalance can cause a flushing sensation. This is particularly true of the middle of the night sweats, which she felt were more linked to my adrenals pushing out the stress hormones as opposed to "true" menopausal sweats. She explained that eating protein with each meal and having a small bedtime snack would help to keep my sugar levels stable.

'I gradually reduced my coffee and wine intake as recommended rather than simply going cold turkey. I thought it would be really tough cutting the caffeine and alcohol down but once I started the programme it became much easier, plus within the first three weeks there was a marked improvement in my hot flushes and night sweats.

'The small bedtime snack she asked me to incorporate seemed to really help my sleep pattern and I was no longer waking in the early hours feeling hot and sweaty. Because of this my energy was so much better and my mood was more stable.

'I was eating a lot more vegetarian protein including chickpeas, lentils, miso and flaxseeds (linseeds), which are rich in compounds called phytoestrogens. These are very weakly oestrogenic, which means they help to top up oestrogen levels that naturally decline during the menopause. Before the consultation I had never heard of some of these foods, let alone eaten them, but now they are second nature to me.

'Alongside the dietary changes she advised me to take vitamins and minerals and a herbal formula containing black cohosh, agnus castus, dong quai, sage and milk thistle, specifically for the hot flushes and sweats. The improvement in my symptoms was remarkable.

'I now go through the day without having to carry a fan and at night my husband also gets to sleep because I'm not throwing the duvet off or opening a window every hour! Thank you, Marilyn.'

MY APPROACH

This book will help you understand the changes that are taking place in your body during the two stages of the menopause. You will learn how to nourish your body and protect yourself from the various degenerative illnesses listed before. I will teach you the fundamentals of good nutrition with my Twelve-Step Hormone Balancing Diet, which you should aim to adopt no matter what your age or what stage you are at. In addition, I will also give you specific dietary recommendations as I discuss each stage of the menopause. Your diet, along with any supplements I recommend, should give you energy, a healthy weight, optimum mental health and help slow down the ageing process. Think of your diet as the foundation of your health: everything you eat provides your body with the materials to produce hormones, brain chemicals (neurotransmitters) and everything necessary to keep your body running effectively.

By following my plan, you can look forward to a natural menopause journey with the minimum of uncomfortable or debilitating symptoms. My healthcare philosophy is very simple and yet very powerful: my aim is always to allow the body to heal itself. If you nourish your body well by following a healthy diet, adding in nutrients in supplement form and herbs if needed, then any problems really can be rectified. My other aim is to always treat my patients as a 'whole person' because, after all, everything in the body is connected. For example, as my patients start to improve their general health I very often see a 'domino effect' whereby different symptoms in the body, often to do with digestive problems, skin health, energy or joints, will all start to improve, too. It is fascinating to watch and very empowering for my patients.

Of course, medical intervention can be life saving, and it is important to recognise when the nutritional approach should be used and when you should move on to medical help. In my opinion, this is easy with the stages of the menopause because, for women, this is a natural event in our lives that *should* be happening. The menopause is not a medical condition to be treated by replacing hormones with hormone replacement therapy (HRT). This is like saying that Mother Nature has got it wrong, that there is something missing and we need to 'rectify' this by putting those hormones back again.

The menopause is simply a transition, a moving from one stage in our lives to another. Somebody once said that it is like going through puberty backwards. We would not think of treating puberty as a medical condition so why the menopause?

As well as the physical side of your health, it is also important to maintain good emotional health. As I will explain, the adrenal glands

6

(your 'stress' glands) play a large part in the ease with which you go through these different stages. Stress can make the menopause transition harder because it can interfere with the production of female hormones. It can also make you more susceptible to health problems and increase your risk of conditions such as osteoporosis, heart disease and diabetes. It is therefore important to address both the emotional and physical side of your health at each stage of the menopause.

With this in mind, take a moment to think about the changes that lie ahead, or the changes you have already been through, and start to try to approach the menopause journey with an open mind. I want you to learn how to tap into your positive emotions and think of this phase of life as an exciting one, filled with opportunity for you to be in the best health you can be, fighting fit and ready for the future.

HOW THIS BOOK WORKS

Part One gives an overview of the menopause process and covers what you can expect in terms of changes to your hormones. It offers diet and lifestyle guidance for optimum health as you approach the menopause and advice on anti-ageing and general wellbeing. The rest of the book is divided into the two stages of the menopause: peri-menopause (when you 'go through' the menopause – Part Two) and postmenopause (after the menopause – Part Three). Each part will take you through what is happening to your body at that time and the symptoms you may be experiencing. I will explain why symptoms occur and how you can use nutrition and natural remedies to combat them. I will draw your attention to any symptoms that indicate you should see your doctor.

Each stage will cover all those aspects of your health that you might have concerns about, namely digestion, skin, hair, nails, energy levels or weight issues, and highlight where you need to pay particular attention, for example to bone health, heart, urinary tract and vagina. I will also cover the foods that are most important during that stage and what are best to avoid.

In each part, I also cover any medical and nutritional tests that may be useful to have at that particular stage of the menopause, either to pick up a potential problem or that would be useful to help you focus on prevention.

PART ONE

PREPARING YOUR BODY FOR THE MENOPAUSE

CHAPTER 1

WHAT'S GOING ON WITH MY HORMONES?

From around the age of 40 your body will start preparing for the menopause, or the cessation of periods, which will take you into the next third of your life (one-third before puberty, one-third between puberty and the menopause, and one-third in the postmenopause). You will start to experience hormone changes that can give rise to a myriad of symptoms. As these changes happen, it is not unusual for some women to think that they are going 'crazy' during this time, and it is important to know that these effects are common and that you *can* do something about them. The physical symptoms you may start to experience include hot flushes, night sweats, lack of sex drive, tiredness, weight gain, vaginal dryness, drier skin and hair, joint pains, hair loss and headaches. You may also experience psychological symptoms such as depression, mood swings, forgetfulness, lack of concentration, loss of confidence and self-esteem, anxiety and tearfulness.

As women, our health and wellbeing are somewhat dependent on our hormones because they take us on such a roller-coaster ride for most of our lives. We have to have a monthly cycle in order to conceive, and this means we have to ride through the peaks and troughs of hormone changes every month. And then the menopause happens, at which point our hormone levels decline and our bodies move into a different stage altogether.

Men do not experience this same roller-coaster; their hormones tend to stabilise after puberty and continue in a steady manner for the rest of their lives. It is different for women: as our monthly cycle involves intricate changes in hormones, it is easier for things to get out of balance and for us to have more health problems connected to our reproductive system than men. Indeed, when you consider the number of hormonal problems that can affect women, including fibroids, endometriosis, polycystic ovary syndrome, cyclical breast problems,

TREATING YOUR SYMPTOMS

Conventional medicine sees your body as a set of separate systems that operate concurrently. If you have joint pains and see a rheumatologist, they will not be interested in your digestive problems because they would be dealt with by a gastroenterologist. However, your diet may be not only affecting the joints and causing inflammation but also upsetting the bowels. The rheumatologist might prescribe non-steroidal anti-inflammatory drugs (NSAIDs – such as ibuprofen) for the joint pains. These could then go on to aggravate your digestive problems because they irritate the gastrointestinal tract and side effects can include gastrointestinal bleeding, diarrhoea and indigestion (dyspepsia) with heartburn, bloating, belching and nausea. You might then be prescribed drugs to offset the side effects of the NSAIDs, which could give you other side effects.

My approach is always to identify and treat the root cause of a problem, rather than just suppressing the symptoms. With my natural solutions – a combination of nutritional and lifestyle changes – you need never be concerned about unwanted side effects that would worsen your condition.

PMS and period problems (heavy, painful, irregular and no periods), and compare this list with men's hormone problems, prostate issues later in life is about all they might have to face.

The decline of female hormones around the menopause can lead to increased risk of certain illnesses such as osteoporosis and also other changes in our bodies like thinning of the vagina, making intercourse uncomfortable and making us more vulnerable to urinary tract and vaginal infections. It is important to be realistic about the fact that you will experience these and other changes but you should also know that being prepared with knowledge means you can work on prevention or alleviation of those symptoms. It is also important for you to know that you are not alone and that many women are experiencing the same issues.

THE STAGES OF THE MENOPAUSE

There is a lot of confusion around the word 'menopause' and the stages of the menopause. The word menopause comes from the Greek, with '*menos*' meaning month and '*pausos*' an ending. To clarify, the menopause can be broken down into three stages:

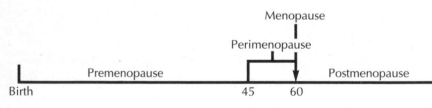

STAGE OF MENOPAUSE TIMELINE

PREMENOPAUSE

The 'premenopause' is often used to describe the whole of a woman's life from her first period to the last one, which usually occurs around the age of 50, but it can happen much earlier for some women and later for others.

PERIMENOPAUSE

When women talk about 'going through the menopause' this is the stage they are really talking about. 'Peri' means 'around', so this is the stage that leads up to the menopause, but sometimes it includes the first 12 months after the last period. This stage can last between two and six years. The actual 'menopause' is the point when you have your last ever period. Obviously you won't know it is your last period until you look back, and you need to have had no periods for 12 months for the menopause to have occurred.

POSTMENOPAUSE

This is the rest of your life beyond the menopause, after your last ever period, but is usually only counted from 12 months after the last menstrual cycle, as it is only known it is the last one once a year has gone by.

THE ROLE YOUR HORMONES PLAY

Hormones play an incredibly important role in your body and can affect your mood and health, now and in the future.

I am now going to explain in detail how the female cycle works and the role of the female hormones so that it is easier to see what is happening to your body as you go through the different stages of the menopause.

THE MENSTRUAL CYCLE

A number of glands and hormones are involved in a female cycle and each phase of the cycle is dependent on the previous phase functioning normally.

During the first half of the menstrual cycle – the follicular phase – FSH (follicle stimulating hormone) is released from the pituitary gland situated at the base of the brain. As the name suggests, FSH stimulates follicles on the ovaries to grow and it is these follicles that contain eggs.

Over approximately the next 14 days the eggs inside the follicles grow and mature. While this is happening, the ovaries are producing increasing amounts of oestrogen. As the oestrogen level increases, so FSH production decreases and another hormone, LH (luteinising hormone), is produced by the pituitary gland. LH is released with a 'surge' and it is this surge that tells the ovaries to release the most mature egg from one of the follicles.

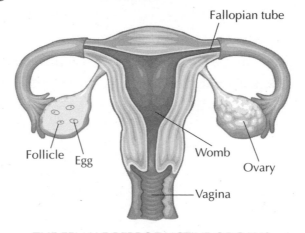

THE FEMALE REPRODUCTIVE ORGANS

Once the egg is released (ovulation) it is literally caught by the Fallopian tube and starts its journey down to the womb (uterus). At the same time that this is happening, the empty follicle (now called the corpus luteum) starts to produce the hormone progesterone.

As soon as ovulation has taken place, the second phase of the cycle, the luteal phase, begins. One of two situations happens at this point: if the egg is fertilised, which happens in the Fallopian tube, it will arrive at the womb as an embryo and implant in the endometrium, the lining of the womb. The level of progesterone continues to rise as it will hold the developing baby in place for approximately the first 12 weeks until the placenta takes over.

If fertilisation does *not* happen, the lining of the womb starts to break down and is shed from the body as the period. Both oestrogen and progesterone production drop and the body is ready to start the next cycle. The first day of the period is also the first day of the next hormone cycle and then it starts all over again, so there are constant hormonal upheavals taking place in your body.

Although we generally talk about a woman's cycle being 28 days long, cycles can vary from 23 to 35 days. As long as your cycle length is approximately the same each month, that is fine. It only becomes a problem if your cycle is such that you could not predict within a day or so when the period would come.

One last point regarding ovulation; most women tend to think of ovulation happening on the fourteenth day of the cycle (with the first day of the period being day one), but in fact ovulation usually happens 14 to 16 days *before* the period so, in a 33-day cycle, ovulation may not take place until day 19. There can also be cycles when you do not ovulate but still have a period. This will be more common as you get closer to the menopause and will be discussed in Part Two.

AN OVERVIEW OF FEMALE HORMONES

There are a number of hormones that we think of as largely 'female', which are also produced in men albeit in different quantities. All of these 'steroid hormones', as they are known, use cholesterol as their starting point.

Oestrogen

Oestrogen is known as the 'female hormone', although men do also produce the same hormone, just in lesser amounts. It is the hormone that causes our breasts to develop during puberty and gives us our womanly shape. Surprisingly, oestrogen is made from male hormones.

Although we talk about oestrogen, there is not actually one single hormone called oestrogen. Your body produces three different oestrogens called oestradiol, oestrone and oestriol. *Oestradiol* is the 'strongest' oestrogen and is produced by the ovary; it is the dominant form from puberty to the menopause. *Oestriol* is the main oestrogen during pregnancy, produced by the placenta. At the menopause, *oestrone* is then produced by the adrenal glands and oestrogen-manufacturing fat cells.

As well as helping develop our sexual characteristics through puberty, oestrogen has other functions including helping to thicken the womb lining ready for a pregnancy, increasing vaginal lubrication, thickening the vaginal wall, increasing bone formation and reducing bone loss, skin health, increasing HDL (or 'good' cholesterol) and decreasing LDL (or 'bad' cholesterol), as well as helping to lift one's mood.

Progesterone

Progesterone is produced in the ovaries by the corpus luteum, the structure that is left after the egg has been released at ovulation. It is a key hormone in pregnancy. Progesterone is also produced by the adrenal glands as well as by the placenta during pregnancy. This hormone helps to maintain a pregnancy by preparing the placenta for implantation and it also prevents further fertilisation by making the vaginal mucus hostile to sperm. It is also the hormone that triggers the menstrual bleed when the level decreases in the second half of the cycle because pregnancy has not occurred.

During the perimenopause there will be cycles where you are not ovulating but could still be having a period so your progesterone levels will be low. This will continue into the menopause and beyond.

Testosterone (androgens)

From puberty, both the ovaries and adrenal glands produce male hormones. The levels of androgens, or male hormones, can decline in women from the age of 40, giving symptoms such as loss of libido and lack of energy. Levels of testosterone for women in their forties can be half those of women in their twenties.[1] Although testosterone production from the ovaries declines, it is not such a dramatic drop as happens with oestrogen at the menopause. Unfortunately for women who have their ovaries removed their testosterone levels will fall suddenly and this can affect their sex drive.

OVARIAN RESERVE (YOUR EGG SUPPLY)

A woman is born with her complete supply of eggs. By around the fifth month of pregnancy, a female foetus can have as many as 7 million eggs, and yet by the time she is born that reserve will have already dropped to around 2 million. At puberty she will have around 750,000, by 45 the number has dropped rapidly to around 10,000 and at the menopause the supply runs out.

The menopause occurs when you do not have enough eggs left in the ovaries to ovulate. To try and get you to ovulate, your body produces more of the follicle stimulating hormone (FSH) to try and trigger ovulation, but that can't happen because the egg supply is too low. Your body will then produce even more FSH to try again. (It is this hormone that provides one way of testing whether you have started going through menopause. A blood test that shows excess FSH, combined with other tests, could confirm that you have.)

CHAPTER 2

MY TWELVE-STEP HORMONE BALANCING DIET

Your diet forms the very foundation of your health. What you eat and drink is the fuel that feeds the biochemical processes in your body, which then uses the nutrients you consume to manufacture hormones to give you energy, to feed your skin, hair and nails, and keep you alive. In the same way that you would not dream of putting poor quality fuel in a very expensive car, you should treat your body with respect. Your body is the vehicle that takes you through life so you need to treat it well and provide the right nutrition to help prevent certain illnesses such as cancer, heart disease, osteoporosis and diabetes.

THE FOUNDATIONS OF GOOD HEALTH

Research has shown that changing the diet can reduce the risk of a number of cancers that are driven by oestrogen, including breast cancer,[1] womb (endometrial) cancer[2] and ovarian cancer.[3] In fact, according to the World Cancer Research Fund in 2009, 40 per cent of all cancers could be prevented by changes in diet and lifestyle, and only 5 per cent are actually due to a genetic disposition.

As well as ensuring that you eat a good diet, nutritional medicine involves making sure that any vitamin, mineral, essential fatty acids or other deficiencies are corrected using food supplements. It also involves ensuring that your digestive system is working efficiently so that the good food can be absorbed and used correctly, and that all the waste and toxins are eliminated properly. Care should be taken to make sure that the levels of good bacteria in the gut are sufficient.

The main aim of my nutritional advice is to get you into good health whatever your age and then help you to maintain it. With this in mind, I have developed a special eating plan that will help combat weight gain, menopausal symptoms and disease. My Twelve-Step Hormone Balancing Diet, which is the subject of this chapter, is designed to help get you on track, with healthy guidelines for all women, no matter what your age.

Whatever stage of the menopause you are at, the food you eat should help your body to adjust easily and comfortably to the hormonal changes you are undergoing and help smooth your menopause journey. Your diet can have a big impact on your hormonal health through the stages of the menopause, nourishing your body and helping control and eliminate unwanted menopause symptoms along the way.

THE DIET

During the menopause your female hormones will be fluctuating up and down until you come out the other side and into the post-menopause, when your hormones will stabilise. The more gradually you go through the menopause, the fewer hormone fluctuations you experience and the easier the transition. Maintaining a balanced diet and healthy lifestyle, and reducing stress levels, can play an important role in making this transition smoother. This diet is designed to help balance your hormones and make the process easier on your body.

Summarised below are the key points of my Twelve-Step Hormone Balancing Diet. (Some are particularly important at certain stages of the menopause, and I will explain why on the following pages.)

1. Include hormone-balancing phytoestrogens in your diet.
2. Eat more Omega 3 fatty acids.
3. Increase your intake of fruit and vegetables.
4. Change from refined carbohydrates to unrefined ones.
5. Buy organic foods where possible.
6. Reduce your intake of saturated fat.
7. Make sure you drink enough fluids.
8. Increase your intake of fibre.
9. Eliminate foods containing chemicals from your diet.
10. Avoid or reduce your intake of caffeine.
11. Reduce or eliminate alcohol.
12. Avoid refined sugar.

STEP 1: INCLUDE HORMONE-BALANCING PHYTOESTROGENS IN YOUR DIET

Phytoestrogens are plant foods that can have an oestrogen-like activity and a hormone-balancing effect on your body. They include pulses such as lentils, chickpeas and soya products. Over 300 foods including fruits, vegetables, seeds, legumes and grains have been found to have this oestrogenic effect but there are differences in the type and strength of the phytoestrogens in these different foods.

Phytoestrogens became of interest to scientists when they realised that women in certain traditional cultures like Japan, who eat a diet rich in these plant foods, have fewer menopausal symptoms than Western women,[4] and also a lower incidence of breast cancer, heart disease, osteoporosis. Scientists wanted to learn how these foods were helping and how they can help us in the Western world, too.

Phytoestrogens are really important in helping combat the effects of the perimenopause and the menopause. Put simply, these plant foods help to balance your hormones. They supply you with an oestrogenic 'activity' (where needed), which will help with the symptoms of the menopause such as hot flushes, night sweats and memory changes, but without risking a serious illness such as cancer (see page 175 about HRT). It is helpful to know how they do this so I describe their function in some detail below.

There are three kinds of phytoestrogens:

Isoflavones: Found in high concentrations in legumes such as soya, chickpeas and lentils.

Lignans: The highest amounts are found in flaxseeds (linseeds) but also in other oil seeds (such as sesame and sunflower seeds), cereals (such as rice, oats and wheat) and vegetables (such as broccoli and carrots).

Coumestans: Found in sprouted mung and alfalfa beans.

Isoflavones are particularly important when you are going through the menopause. There are four different types of isoflavones: genistein, daidzein, biochanin and formononetin. What is interesting is that the different legumes contain different ratios of these isoflavones. Soya contains both genistein and daidzein; chickpeas and lentils contain all four. Each of these isoflavones will have different benefits, so variety is the key. I regularly see women in the clinic who are overdoing their intake of soya because they have heard that it is good for them and are therefore eating too much and missing out on the other legumes such as lentils and chickpeas. (For more on soya consumption, see page 25.)

For different cultures around the world, legumes have been a staple part of the diet for centuries. Examples include tofu in Asia, hummus (made from chickpeas) in the Middle East and dhal (made from lentils) in India. Whole families – women, men and children – are brought up on these phytoestrogenic foods. Peas and green beans are types of legumes that we have traditionally eaten in the West, but we do not eat anywhere near the same amount; the average intake for isoflavones in the East is around 45mg per day compared to only 2mg in the West.

The word phytoestrogen can be confusing – how can having 'extra' oestrogen be good for men and how can these foods *lower* the risk of breast cancer for women when we know that excess oestrogen can stimulate breast cancer?

BREAST CANCER RATES

In the West, breast cancer affects 133 women per 100,000 whereas in Asian countries, it is more than three times lower at 39 women per 100,000.

Research has shown that a diet high in soya is associated with a 14 per cent reduction in risk of breast cancer.[5] Two of the best soya foods for breast health are tofu and miso.[6]

Phytoestrogens (isoflavones) literally work like a key. The cells in your body have oestrogen receptors on them that act like a lock; they need a key that fits into that lock to 'stimulate' them into activity. This activity can be beneficial in certain places in the body such as your bones and brain where you want the cells to stay active, but can be negative in other places such as the breasts and womb where you do not want cells to be too stimulated, causing them to multiply and then mutate. There are two different kinds of oestrogen receptors, alpha and beta.

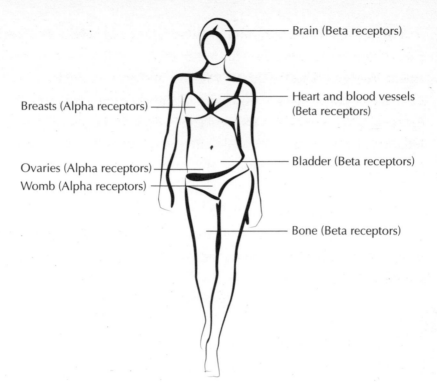

Brain (Beta receptors)

Heart and blood vessels
(Beta receptors)

Breasts (Alpha receptors)

Bladder (Beta receptors)

Ovaries (Alpha receptors)
Womb (Alpha receptors)

Bone (Beta receptors)

OESTROGEN RECEPTORS IN THE FEMALE BODY

You have alpha receptors in your breasts, ovaries and womb and beta receptors in your brain, bones, blood vessels and bladder, as well as in your breasts, ovaries and womb. Your breasts, ovaries and womb therefore have both alpha and beta receptors.

HRT (see chapter 11) triggers both alpha and beta receptors, which is why it can increase the risk of breast, ovarian and womb cancer when it stimulates the cells in those areas.

Isoflavones, as found in chickpeas, lentils and soya, work in a completely different way. They block the alpha receptors in the breasts, ovaries and womb but stimulate the beta receptors in the brain and bones. So at any stage of the menopause they can help protect you from breast, ovary and womb cancers and yet also help keep your brain and bones healthy. Isoflavones can even help to block the foreign oestrogens, called xenoestrogens (see page 103), coming in from the environment and can prevent them from locking on to your cells. Phytoestrogens work exactly like the new drugs that have been developed for menopausal women called SERMs, selective oestrogen – estrogen in America – receptor modulators, (see page 217), which selectively stimulate the receptors in places where you want stimulation, such as your brain and bones, but not in the places where it would be dangerous, such as your breasts.

THE BENEFITS OF PHYTOESTROGENS FOR MEN

We also know that isoflavones can have a beneficial effect on balancing male hormones and the risk of prostate cancer. Prostate cancer is about 30 times higher in Western men compared to men in China, who have more phytoestrogens in their diet.[7] Phytoestrogens can have the same effect as the testosterone-lowering drugs prescribed for prostate cancer and the International Prostate Health Council has stated that soya can prevent the progression of the dormant form of prostate cancer to the more advanced form.[8] For this reason, as you increase your intake of foods rich in isoflavones for your own benefit, your partner may want to increase his, too.

Phytoestrogens also stimulate a protein produced by the liver called SHBG (sex hormone binding globulin) and this protein does exactly what it says it does, binds hormones. It can bind oestrogen (or testosterone in men) and prevent too much circulating in your body. This mirrors the work of anti-oestrogen drugs for certain breast cancers (and the work of testosterone-lowering drugs for prostate cancer).

For isoflavones to give you this beneficial hormone-balancing effect they have to go through a process of fermentation. They should be fermented either in the form of food processing, for example miso, or by the bacteria in your gut. But with people using so many antibiotics nowadays these can effectively 'wipe out' the good bacteria in your gut and people lose the ability to process these isoflavones. That is why as well as the immune benefits it is so important to have good levels of beneficial bacteria.

Maximise the benefits of isoflavones

Most of the research on isoflavones has been on soya but remember that *all* the legumes contain isoflavones so vary your diet with different ones. The recommended amount of isoflavones for women is about 45mg a day. As an example, one serving of tofu (2oz/55g) or 1 pint (600ml) of soya milk will give you about 40mg of isoflavones. For a list of foods containing phytoestrogens see Appendix, page 281.

Soya

There has been quite a lot of press about soya and I know women get very confused about what is and isn't good for them. When media coverage is positive, some women will start eating soya in excess amounts in every form possible, whether it be soya yogurt, TVP (textured vegetable protein) or soya bars. If, on the other hand, some negative press appears, some women stop eating it.

I want to set the record straight here so you know exactly what you should be eating and why. Soya is definitely beneficial for your health, especially during the menopause, and the earlier you can start including phytoestrogens of any kind in your diet the better.

The negative press on soya revolves around the *form* of the soya product; it *does not* apply to all soya. You should aim to eat soya in the same way that it is eaten in traditional cultures, such as in Japan and China, in a less processed form than we often eat it in the West. You need to eat soya products that are made from *whole* soya beans.

In the West, soya products made from highly processed soya protein isolates are common, but we don't know what the effects of eating this highly processed soya are on our bodies; we only know the health benefits of eating soya in its whole form. Make sure you read the ingredients list on the soya products you buy; if you see the words 'soya isolate' or 'soya protein isolate', choose a different brand, as this indicates you are buying a highly processed refined food. Soya isolate powder, which is made in an industrial process, is made up into baby formulas, soya milk, tofu, hydrolysed vegetable protein to be used as flavour enhancers in soups and sauces and into vegetarian proteins (TVP) to taste like meat. Aim to buy organic soya as these products will be not be genetically modified.

Remember to include other isoflavones such as chickpeas, lentils and kidney beans in your diet. For some good, easy recipes that contain these legumes see my cookbook *Healthy Eating for the Menopause* (Kyle Cathie).

The benefits of lignans

I should also mention one of the other kinds of phytoestrogens: lignans. Flaxseeds (linseeds) are the richest source of these lignans. Lignans also undergo biotransformation in your digestive system, with the help of good bacteria, into compounds (enterolactone and entero-diol), which have a balancing effect on oestrogen. Their fibre content is also helpful in removing excess oestrogens out through the bowels.[9] The beneficial effect of lignans is increased if you crush or mill the flaxseeds, which you can then sprinkle on porridge or natural yogurt, for example. It is worth pointing out that you do not get the benefits of lignans from flaxseed oil.

A pilot study in 2007 by the Mayo Clinic has suggested that adding 4 tablespoons (40g) of crushed flaxseeds to the daily diet for six weeks can help to reduce the main symptoms of the menopause, namely hot flushes and night sweats, by a half.

I believe it is important to understand how phytoestrogens actually work because it takes away the fear that they could be giving you too much oestrogen. They can't, as you have seen, because they don't work like that.

Q&A

I am taking HRT so will I benefit from eating phytoestrogens?

Including phytoestrogens in your diet may help to offset some of the possible negative side effects of taking HRT, for example the risk of breast cancer, by blocking the receptors in the breast and preventing the powerful oestradiol from the HRT 'locking on'.

I have already had breast cancer and am worried about eating phytoestrogens – is it safe to do so?

You should definitely include these foods in your diet, particularly if your breast cancer was oestrogen receptor positive. You are aiming to work on preventing a recurrence, and as these foods can help prevent breast cells being stimulated by oestrogen then they are beneficial for you. Make sure you eat them in the most natural, unprocessed form possible – as described in this section.

STEP 2: EAT MORE OMEGA 3 FATTY ACIDS

Along with phytoestrogens, I cannot stress enough the importance of including foods that contain essential fatty acids in your diet. Omega 3 fatty acids are found in oily fish such as sardines, salmon, mackerel and also in flaxseeds (linseeds).

It has become more and more evident during my years working in nutrition that when considering essential fatty acid intake, the emphasis must be on the Omega 3 oils and not the Omega 6 variety.

Your body produces substances called prostaglandins from the essential fatty acids, some of which are anti-inflammatory and some of which are pro-inflammatory (meaning they cause inflammation). You may wonder why you would ever want your body to produce inflammation but it is important at the appropriate time. For example, when your body is under attack from bacteria or you have cut yourself, you need your body to react quickly and create heat, pain, soreness, redness even, to make the blood clot faster as it mobilises your immune system to either attack the bacteria or start healing the cut. This is a positive example of 'inflammation'.

What you *don't* want is chronic, persistent inflammation going on in your body, as that can lead to not only visible signs such as joint pains, arthritis, swollen gums and colitis, but also serious illnesses such as heart disease, diabetes, osteoporosis and cancer.

In a nutshell, you want your body to produce more of the anti-inflammatory prostaglandins and less of the pro-inflammatory ones. This is where including Omega 3 fatty acids in your diet is crucial, as they are powerful anti-inflammatories. Over the last century there has been an 80 per cent decrease in the consumption of these Omega 3

ARE YOU GETTING ENOUGH OMEGA 3 FATTY ACIDS?

What many women think of as symptoms connected to the menopause can actually be related to not having enough essential Omega 3 fatty acids. Omega 3 deficiency symptoms can include:

- dry, lifeless hair
- soft, easily frayed nails
- painful joints
- arthritis
- cracked skin on heels or fingertips
- depression and mood swings
- poor wound healing
- dry skin
- difficulty losing weight
- lack of motivation
- fatigue.

fatty acids,[10] which are found mainly in oily fish and oils, flaxseeds and also soya. The trouble is that many people are also eating too much Omega 6 fat, found in vegetable oils, ready meals, fast food, margarine and snacks such as chips, crisps and biscuits.

Omega 3s vs Omega 6s

It is estimated that we are getting ten times more Omega 6 fats from our diet than Omega 3. Many of the women I see in the clinic have been taking evening primrose oil supplements – an Omega 6 fatty acid – for years and have not been eating enough Omega 3 oils, or taking them in supplement form, to counterbalance this (see 'The role of essential fatty acids' below for why the balance is so important). Some women are also taking combination supplements such as Omega 3, 6 and 9, because they have read that they need a good balance of all the Omega fatty acids. This is true, but you have to take into account what your own levels may be in the first place. It is no good adding in more Omega 6 if you have already got enough or even too much in your body. (You can now have a blood test to tell you if you have the correct levels of Omega 3 to Omega 6 in your body – for more information see Useful Resources at the end of the book.)

The role of essential fatty acids

It is useful to have a look at what happens when you eat essential fatty acids. As you can see from the pathway table on page 31, when you eat Omega 6 fats they can *either* be converted to anti-inflammatory (good) or pro-inflammatory (bad) prostaglandins. When you eat Omega 3 fats, they can only ever be converted to the anti-inflammatory substances, which is why having enough of the Omega 3 essential fats is *so* important.

What decides whether the Omega 6 fats get converted to good or bad prostaglandins? First of all, as you eat these essential fats your body converts them into more complex forms. You need good levels of the minerals zinc, magnesium and vitamin B6 to help convert these essential fats. However, the conversion can be blocked by substances such as alcohol and saturated fats. This conversion is also blocked by stress.

Omega 3 fats start off as alpha linolenic acid (ALA) as found in flaxseeds (linseeds), pumpkin, soya and walnuts and your body converts them to EPA (eicosapentaenoic acid) and DHA (docosahexenoic acid) as found naturally in oily fish such as salmon, sardines, mackerel and tuna. The EPA and DHA produce the anti-inflammatory prostaglandins and also help to reduce the pro-inflammatory ones.

Omega 6 fats start off as linoleic acid (LA) found in nuts, seeds and legumes, which is then converted by your body into gamma linolenic acid (GLA), found naturally in evening primrose oil and borage oil. This GLA can then be converted into anti-inflammatory prostaglandins.

But, and this is a big 'but', if you have higher levels of insulin from blood sugar fluctuations or not enough EPA in your system, your body can convert the GLA into arachidonic acid (AA), which produces inflammatory substances. Arachidonic acid is also found naturally in animal foods such as red meat and dairy products.

These inflammatory substances not only cause pain, such as from arthritis, but they also make your blood clot faster thus increasing the risk of heart disease. The inflammation can also cause skin problems such as eczema.

If you have high levels of insulin and your body stops the conversion of GLA into good anti-inflammatory prostaglandins this produces more inflammation. This inflammation in turn stops your body responding efficiently to insulin, so it tries to compensate by making yet more insulin, which in turn causes more inflammation and leaves you stuck in a vicious cycle.

It is really not good to take GLA supplements such as evening primrose oil if you have blood sugar fluctuations because the higher levels of insulin caused by this roller-coaster are going to make your body produce more inflammation.

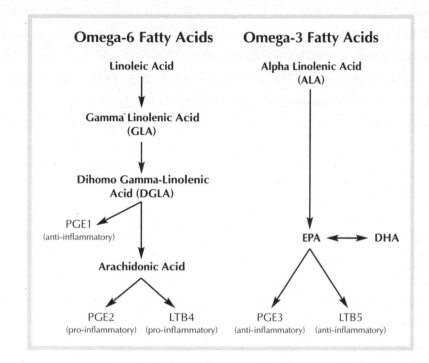

OMEGA 6 AND OMEGA 3 PATHWAYS

As you can see from the diagram, your body produces the good, anti-inflammatory prostaglandins directly from EPA and DHA, which are contained in *oily fish*. If you are a vegetarian then your body has to convert the ALA from flaxseeds or soya, for example, into EPA and DHA. Unfortunately, it is estimated that only about 10 per cent of the ALA gets converted when everything is ideal, but if you are stressed, drinking too much alcohol or not getting enough key nutrients (particularly zinc, magnesium and vitamin B6) your conversion rate will probably be even less than 10 per cent.

STEP 3: INCREASE YOUR INTAKE OF FRUIT AND VEGETABLES

Fruit and vegetables are your anti-ageing foods. They contain antioxidants, which are a group of vitamins, minerals and unique compounds with incredible health benefits for women during all the stages of the menopause. They fight the damaging effects of free radicals – nasty substances produced by simple body functions, such as breathing, the way you cook your food, such as barbecuing, and lifestyle habits, such as smoking, that can wreak havoc at a cellular level and make you more susceptible to heart disease, weight gain, cancer and signs of premature ageing (wrinkles). These free radicals can damage healthy cells thus speeding up the ageing process but they can also cause cell mutations, which can lead to cancer.

Fortunately, antioxidants are found in many foods. Foods rich in vitamins C, E and beta-carotene (the plant form of vitamin A) all have antioxidant properties, as do foods rich in the minerals selenium and zinc. Some important plant chemicals are also antioxidants, for example lycopene (found in tomatoes), bioflavonoids (found in citrus fruits) and proanthocyanins (found in berries and grapes).

The aim is to at eat least five servings of antioxidant fruit and vegetables a day. But the UK National Diet and Nutrition Survey in 2008/9 found that only a third of men and women are eating the recommended 'five-a-day' fruit and vegetables, and according to the UK Food Standards Agency the average consumption of fruit and vegetables is fewer than three servings a day.

Targets in other countries are very different from those in the UK. In the US the recommendation is to eat between five and 13 portions of fruit and vegetables a day. In Australia they recommend seven and specify that this is made up from five vegetables and two fruit. Japan is aiming even higher with a total of 17 (13 vegetables and four fruit). It is thought that the UK government settled on five a day as the amount they thought we could manage, but unfortunately we are not even achieving that. Try not to focus on 'five a day' as your goal, but rather your starting point!

To get good levels of different antioxidants aim to 'eat a rainbow'. My mother always talked about 'eating our greens', but we now know that all the different colours in the fruit and vegetables give us different antioxidants, which have beneficial effects on our health. Think of colourful fruits such as blueberries, raspberries, apples and tomatoes, and the wide variety of colourful vegetables such as sweetcorn, green vegetables, beetroot, pumpkin (squash) and carrots all available at your local supermarket or farmers' market.

Try out some new recipes and aim to include at least one new vegetable and fruit in your diet each week. You can experiment with snacking on fruit pieces, adding some to an organic natural yogurt at breakfast or including different types of fruits in a smoothie. Another good way to experiment with different vegetables is to use them in a soup; this is also a good way to get in more of your five a day.

STEP 4: CHANGE FROM REFINED CARBOHYDRATES TO UNREFINED ONES

Carbohydrates are an important part of your diet as they give you energy, but it is the *type* of carbohydrate you consume that determines the *quality* of that energy, that is, whether it is short- or long-lasting.

There is a lot of confusion around carbohydrates so my aim is to make this section really clear. Everybody thinks of carbohydrates as being starchy foods such as rice, pasta, bread and potatoes, but vegetables such as broccoli are also carbohydrates.

Refined carbohydrates vs unrefined carbohydrates

In a nutshell, carbohydrates are sugars and starches. There are two kinds of carbohydrates – simple and complex. What is important is whether they are *refined* or *unrefined*. When a carbohydrate is refined, the fibre and a lot of the goodness is stripped away, so when you eat a food containing refined carbohydrates that food will cause glucose to be released into your bloodstream quickly.

This is the theory behind the glycemic index (GI), which is a measurement of how quickly or slowly a food releases glucose into the bloodstream. Carbohydrates are ranked according to their GI value and glucose is given a glycemic index of 100. All carbohydrates are broken down into glucose when you eat them and the index measures how quickly or slowly they do that. All carbohydrates are then compared to the GI of glucose. The more refined a food, the higher the glycemic index will be. You can also slow the release of glucose from a carbohydrate by eating it with a protein (either vegetable or animal).

Simple carbohydrates include fruit, sugar and honey. They are called 'simple' because they have a simple molecular structure, compared to the complex carbohydrates, and this simple structure means they are absorbed more quickly. Simple carbohydrates can be refined (white and brown sugar) or unrefined (fruit). The same is true for complex carbohydrates. This group includes grains, beans and vegetables. Again, complex carbohydrates can be refined and the fibre removed (such as in white bread and white rice) or unrefined where all the fibre and a lot of the valuable nutrients have been retained, such as in brown rice, wholemeal bread or wholewheat pasta). The table below tells you which foods are refined and unrefined carbohydrates:

UNREFINED	REFINED
Barley	Biscuits, cakes and pastries
Beans and pulses	made with white flour and
Brown rice	sugar
Buckwheat (part of rhubarb family)	Breakfast cereals with added
Fruit (particularly berries, apples	sugar
and pears and citrus)	Brown and white sugar
Maize	Fruit juice (as the fibre has
Millet	been removed)
Nuts	Instant 'quick cook' porridge
Oats	oats

UNREFINED	REFINED
Rye	Soft fizzy drinks
Spelt	Treacle
Vegetables	White bread
Wholemeal breads	White flour
Wholemeal flour	White rice
Wholewheat pasta	

You want to be eating unrefined carbohydrates (simple or complex) not just because they provide more valuable nutrients, but because, most importantly, they supply good slow-release energy throughout the day, enabling you to avoid the highs and lows of blood sugar surges. This is important as you go through the menopause because your moods may be fluctuating due to hormonal changes and being on a roller-coaster of blood sugar swings will only make this worse. Also, as you will see on page 50, when your blood sugar drops your adrenal glands release stress hormones. At the menopause, your adrenal glands need to produce a form of oestrogen to help protect your bones (as the production of oestrogen from the ovaries declines). You don't want to overwork your adrenal glands while they do this, as their production of oestrogen could be lessened, so protect yourself from blood sugar dips and they won't be prompted to release stress hormones.

STEP 5: BUY ORGANIC FOODS WHERE POSSIBLE

From a health perspective, there are two reasons to buy organic food: one is that these foods are likely to contain more valuable nutrients because they are grown on soil that is not depleted; the other important reason is that you are reducing your exposure to xenoestrogens (see page 103), which come from the pesticide and plastic industries. At this time in your life, when your body is going through a hormonal transition, you do not want to upset that delicate balance by exposing yourself to unnecessary excessive amounts of external oestrogen. Also, excess oestrogens are a risk factor for breast cancer, so buy organic food where your budget allows so that you can reduce the risk.

If you are on a tight budget, try to buy the smallest foods as organic. The smaller the food, the more pesticide it can absorb, so, for example, choose organic grains, such as wholemeal bread, rice and oats instead of larger vegetables such as sweet potatoes, which can be peeled. Also, the more fragile the fruit or vegetable the more it will be sprayed with pesticides in order to protect it. Lettuces and berries may be sprayed numerous times before they reach the supermarket shelves. I also recommend that you invest in organic dairy products and eggs because organic feed given to the animals that produce them is going to give you more nutritional benefits from the products that you eat.

STEP 6: REDUCE YOUR INTAKE OF SATURATED FAT

Saturated fats are found in animal products such as meat and dairy and are also found in tropical oils such as palm oil. Unfortunately, high levels of saturated fat in your diet increase the level of oestrogen in your blood.[11] You might think having extra oestrogen would be useful at this stage in your life as your own levels of this hormone are decreasing, but excess oestrogen can increase your risk of breast cancer so it is better to reduce your intake of saturated fat.

Saturated fat also contains arachidonic acid (AA), which causes your body to produce more inflammation (see page 31), and this fat can also interfere with your Omega 3 and Omega 6 fat levels, making it harder for your body to use them in a healthy and efficient way.

The standard thinking is that 'saturated fats make you fat' but I will blow this myth apart in the section on weight management (page 147). I also don't think that saturated fat increases cholesterol or, in fact, that cholesterol is the 'baddy' it is made out to be – this is explored in more detail on page 226.

Use saturated fat in moderation. I will choose organic butter instead of margarine, for example, as I think it is a more natural product, but use it sparingly.

The real fat 'baddy' – trans fats

I need to mention one other kind of fat that is worse than saturated fat and that is *trans fat*. Trans fats are found in many processed foods (such as cakes and biscuits), fast foods and also margarines. Trans fats are produced by chemically altering liquid oils to make them into solids by passing hydrogen through the oil at a high temperature and under pressure (or 'hydrogenating' the oil). Trans fats can also occur naturally in some foods, such as milk, but the amount is negligible. Trans fats do not have to be listed in the nutritional information on a food label or in the ingredient list, but if a food label says 'hydrogenated vegetable oil' then it can contain trans fats.

The value of trans fats to the food industry is enormous as they are cheap and extend shelf life for years, while liquid oils can go rancid fairly quickly. But trans fats have no nutritional benefit whatsoever and are in fact detrimental to your health as they can increase your risk of heart disease. They also increase bad cholesterol (LDL) and decrease good cholesterol (HDL). Research has shown that by increasing your consumption of trans fats by just 2 per cent you can increase your risk of heart disease by 30 per cent.[12] Trans fats can also block the absorption of essential fatty acids, create more inflammation in your body and stop the production of beneficial anti-inflammatory substances.

Although trans fats are unsaturated fats they are *worse* than saturated fats because they act like a plastic in your body, which attempts to use them as if they are essential fatty acids, meaning they can end up in cell membranes. These trans fats harden cells causing them to lose their elasticity, which is bad news for blood vessels and for your heart. Trans fats can also harden cells by affecting insulin receptors, making you more resistant to insulin and putting you at risk of Type 2 diabetes.

In addition, your brain is 70 per cent fat, but it has to be the right type of fat and brain cells need to be flexible to function properly. Consuming trans fats can make your mental functions such as memory and concentration less efficient. An interesting study was done on children, where the researchers found that those children who ate margarine daily had IQ scores up to six points lower compared to children who did not. Fish consumption on the other hand boosted intelligence.[13]

No matter what age you are, you want to make sure that your brain is functioning well. You cannot blame everything on age when there can be other factors that determine how well you think and remember – especially through this stage in your life.

In 2003 Denmark was the first country to ban the sale of foods containing more than 2 per cent trans fat, which means they have banned partially hydrogenated oils altogether (because they will contain more than 2 per cent). This ban covers the ingredients rather than the final food product, which is excellent news. In 2008, Switzerland followed suit and trans fats are also now banned in New York and Austria, and hopefully more countries, including the UK, will fall in line.

I suggest you avoid trans fats completely and shun products where the ingredients label includes hydrogenated or partially hydrogenated oils.

STEP 7: MAKE SURE YOU ARE DRINKING ENOUGH FLUIDS

Your body is two-thirds water, which provides the means for nutrients to travel to organs and for toxins to be removed from them. In addition, water helps your body metabolise stored fat, making it crucial for weight management. With regard to drinking water, one question I am often asked in the clinic is 'How much is enough?' There is no easy answer to this one! The usual recommendation is to drink at least 2½ pints/1.5 litres (six to eight glasses) of water a day. (I recommend that you drink filtered tap water or mineral water from glass bottles.) It has been suggested that this volume should be calculated on the size of the person, taking their weight in pounds and halving it to see how much water (in fluid ounces) should be drunk in a day, but even this is not so helpful, because the need for water depends on so many factors.

Water is lost through urination, respiration and sweating, and symptoms of mild dehydration include joint pain, irritability, headache, tension, swollen ankles and a bloated stomach. If your urine has a strong odour and is yellow or amber in colour, this can be an indicator of dehydration, as well as the obvious sign of thirst (although in fact often the body needs water long before it registers it is thirsty).

You need to increase your water intake if you drink tea, coffee, alcohol and caffeinated fizzy drinks as these can dehydrate the body. Intake should also be increased if you are exercising a lot, travelling by plane, eating a lot of salty foods or spending time in a hot climate.

Don't think you can only drink plain water though; non-caffeinated herbal teas count towards your daily fluid intake too as they are not dehydrating (unlike caffeinated beverages). Water served hot or cold with a slice of lemon can help ring the changes. Water down fruit juices so they are not too concentrated. Remember, if you are eating a good amount of fruit and vegetables, you do not need quite as much extra fluid as these can contain up to 90 per cent water.

If you enjoy sparkling mineral water it is fine in moderation, but choose the naturally sparkling type (look on the label), otherwise the carbon dioxide added to make the water sparkling can cause flatulence.

STEP 8: INCREASE YOUR INTAKE OF FIBRE

Most people know that fibre is good for the bowels, which it is, but not everyone knows there are two forms of fibre (insoluble and soluble), which have different effects on your body as you eat them. Foods can contain both soluble and insoluble fibre but they are usually classified according to the most dominant fibre in that food.

It is the *insoluble fibre* that affects your bowels because it helps the stools to be bulky and soft. This type of fibre is found in whole grains and vegetables.

The *soluble fibre* found in oats, beans and fruit plays a role in controlling cholesterol because it binds with the cholesterol from your food and helps to excrete it.

In 2007, the British Nutrition Foundation listed the nutritional benefits of fibre, which included not only preventing constipation but also reducing the risk of colon cancer, improving blood sugar balance, helping to improve digestive health, reducing high cholesterol and high blood pressure and helping with weight loss by giving a sense of fullness and satisfaction. These are a few of the good reasons why you should up your fibre intake!

Fibre and oestrogen

Another important role played by fibre at this stage in your life is in the control of oestrogen. It may seem strange to think about the digestive system when it comes to balancing hormones but the fibre you eat helps your body excrete 'old' oestrogens out through the bowels. Research from the US National Institutes of Health on diet and cancer has shown that as dietary fibre intake increases so levels of oestrogen decrease. This detoxification of 'old' oestrogen is important because it is effectively what your body has finished with and is aiming to excrete. If it does not do this efficiently, then the oestrogen can recirculate, giving you higher levels of this hormone than you should have and the possible increased risk of breast cancer.

Bran is not the answer

Fibre is a valuable part of your diet, which is why Step 4 of my Twelve-Step Hormone Balancing Diet is so important because by including unrefined carbohydrates in your diet you are naturally including fibre without even thinking about it.

What I am *not* suggesting, however, is that you start by simply adding fibre such as bran to your food. Bran is actually a refined food; it is what has been stripped away to get white flour, for example. If you think about it in that sense, it does seem illogical to then add it back into your diet when you could just eat wholegrain cereals instead. Also, wheat bran can be quite harsh on the digestive system, causing more bloating and irritable bowel symptoms. In addition, most of the high-bran breakfast cereals are actually very high in sugar, which is, in turn, not good for your health (see Step 12).

I recommend that you eat plenty of whole grains, fruits and vegetables to get all the fibre you need in its most natural form.

STEP 9: ELIMINATE FOODS CONTAINING CHEMICALS FROM YOUR DIET

You want your body to go through the different stages of the menopause easily, comfortably and as naturally as possible. Obviously, the more chemicals that are allowed to impact on your body the harder it has to work to deal with these 'foreign' substances, and so fewer resources are available to take you through this transition and keep your hormones balanced as you go through each stage.

In order to keep things as simple as possible for your body, you should make an effort to reduce the amount of man-made chemicals and processed ingredients you inflict on it by reading food labels and choosing foods that do not contain preservatives, artificial flavours, colours or sweeteners. Look for equivalent products that do not contain these chemicals or choose a different product altogether.

Artificial sweeteners – not so sweet?

Watch out for artificial sweeteners in particular. These can be found in many products that are labelled 'no sugar', 'low sugar' or even 'diet'. They can lead to mood swings and depression, and it has been found that these sweeteners can increase your appetite and make you gain weight.[14] When you think that many women use artificial sweeteners to avoid sugar and control their weight it does seem ironic that they may be causing more weight problems than they are solving.

Artificial sweeteners contain fewer calories than sugar; however the issue is not with the calories but the effect they have on the body once they have been consumed. The sweetener confuses your body in the following way: when you taste something sweet, your body expects a certain amount of calories to accompany that food, but because the artificial sweeteners don't actually contain any calories your body can actually make you crave *more* sugary carbohydrate-type foods to feed you the 'missing' calories.

I recommend that you avoid artificial sweeteners completely as I don't believe they are a healthy choice, no matter how good they may be for the food industry because they cost much less to use than natural sweeteners.

See Step 12 for tips on alternatives to refined sugar. Don't be fooled into thinking that brown sugar is better than white; it is usually white sugar with colour added so the effect on your bloodstream and the release of insulin is just the same.

Additives and preservatives

By avoiding additives and preservatives, you are reducing the chemical, toxic load on your body and making it easier for your body to use its resources to go through the hormonal transition of the menopause rather than devoting energy to detoxifying external substances absorbed through your food and drinks. Manufacturers may claim that one particular additive or preservative is safe, especially in small amounts, but nobody knows what the effect of a cocktail of these substances is, especially when they may be contained in a number of foods and drinks that we consume.

My advice, then, is to read the labels and avoid them completely.

STEP 10: AVOID OR REDUCE YOUR INTAKE OF CAFFEINE

Caffeine is found in food and drinks, primarily in chocolate, caffeinated soft drinks, energy drinks, coffee and tea (black, green and white). The problem with caffeine as you go through the different stages of the menopause is that it can make your symptoms worse. Caffeine is a stimulant, which activates your adrenal (stress) glands, and as your adrenal glands are going to produce a form of oestrogen to help protect your bones as you go through the menopause, you do not want to overwork them. Caffeine causes a quick rise in blood sugar so contributes to fluctuating blood sugar swings, which can not only affect your energy but also your moods. And it can also cause your blood vessels to expand making you sweat more, which can increase the hot flushes.

Caffeine also has a diuretic effect, which means you can lose important vitamins and minerals through having too much of it. It also causes an acidic effect on the body, which means that calcium will be lost through your urine at a time when calcium is vital to your bone health.

CAFFEINE CONTENT OF DIFFERENT DRINKS* AND CHOCOLATE

Coffee, filtered	120mg
Coffee, instant	66mg
Tea, ordinary black	60mg
Colas	45–50mg
Chocolate, dark (1oz/28g)	20mg
Tea, green	15mg
Tea, white	15mg
Cocoa	14mg
Chocolate, milk (1oz/28g)	6mg
Coffee, decaffeinated	5mg

(*Caffeine content for drinks is based on a 236ml/8fl oz serving. These values are approximate as, especially with coffee, they can depend on the variety of the bean.)

Caffeine has an addictive effect on the body so if you decide to eliminate it, it is better to wean yourself off rather than go cold turkey, otherwise you can get severe withdrawal effects such as headaches and muscle cramps. You can switch to decaffeinated coffee but coffee contains three stimulants – caffeine, theobromine and theophylline – so even though the caffeine may be less, the other two stimulants are still there. It is a good idea to eliminate it from your diet completely (even decaff) or just keep it for the weekend.

Black tea only contains caffeine, not the other stimulants that coffee has, but it also contains tannin. When you drink a cup of ordinary tea with your food, the tannin will block the absorption of minerals such as calcium, magnesium and iron. If you are drinking black tea then use decaffeinated and don't drink it at the same time as eating, but leave half-an-hour either side of having food.

Unfortunately, chemicals are often used to remove caffeine from tea and coffee so decaffeinated drinks are not recommended on a regular basis since you are aiming to reduce the toxic load on your body as you go through this stage in your life.

You could try coffee substitutes such as grain coffee instead and also try herb teas such as peppermint and chamomile. There is also a South African tea called rooibos (red bush), which naturally grows without caffeine so can be a good alternative to ordinary black tea.

Breast tenderness

If you are still having periods and finding that your breasts are very uncomfortable then it is a good idea to eliminate any foods or drinks containing caffeine from your diet. Certain substances called methylxanthines, found in any food or drink that contains caffeine, have been associated with causing painful, lumpy breasts. Methylxanthines do not affect all women but it is definitely worthwhile eliminating caffeine and seeing whether this makes a difference for you.

STEP 11: REDUCE OR ELIMINATE ALCOHOL

Through the stages of the menopause your body is going through a hormonal transition and the overall aim is to make this as smooth as possible. The organ that deals with the detoxification of hormones is your liver and alcohol is toxic to the liver, and you do not want to put an extra burden on this organ at any stage.

Alcohol is a diuretic, which makes you pass more urine more frequently and can leave you feeling dehydrated. It also acts as an anti-nutrient and blocks the effect of valuable nutrients such as the B vitamins, zinc, calcium and magnesium. Alcohol will also block the conversion of the essential fatty acids (see Step 2 on page 27) and you can then end up producing more inflammatory substances.

The effects of alcohol on your liver

The biggest impact alcohol can have on your body, however, is its effect on your liver. The liver is the largest organ in your body (not counting your skin) and is the only organ that can be cut in half and left to regrow, so incredible are its powers of regeneration.

Alcohol is classed as a hepatoxin, meaning that it is toxic to your liver. Alcohol is a drug and its main ingredient is ethanol, which is absorbed into the bloodstream quickly. As your liver cannot store alcohol, it has to break it down (metabolise it) in order to get rid of it. So, while it can manage small amounts of alcohol, say, one unit an hour, if you drink more than that it simply cannot break it down fast enough. As the liver metabolises alcohol it stores fat in your liver, which over time can lead to fatty liver disease.

Your liver plays many important roles, including helping to balance blood sugar, the production of substances that help your blood to clot, fat metabolism, the production of cholesterol and protein metabolism. In fact, 80 per cent of the body's cholesterol is produced by your liver and only 20 per cent comes from your food, so if your liver is not functioning properly it can end up producing more cholesterol. (Statins are drugs that treat this by blocking the production of cholesterol from the liver.)

You can't live without your liver so it pays not to risk harming it. If, until now, you have been drinking alcohol regularly (even one glass every night) and/or heavily then it is better to take a complete break for about four weeks. After this, I suggest you drink in moderation – only one glass at a time, and always leave a day or so in between so that your liver gets a break. Remember that your liver has only a certain capacity to detoxify, so while it is detoxifying alcohol it has fewer resources to detoxify all the other substances you may be exposed to (such as pollutants, xenoestrogens, additives, preservatives and artificial sweeteners). Lift the burden of work that your body has to do and it will have more energy and resources to heal itself and keep you healthy now and in the long term.

Alcohol and hormones

As well as for your general health, the other reason for keeping alcohol to a minimum or even eliminating it completely at this stage in your life is the effect on your hormones, particularly oestrogen.

Your hard-working liver deactivates oestradiol and oestrone into oestriol (a less harmful form of oestrogen) for it to be eliminated from your body. Your liver also produces a protein called sex hormone binding globulin (SHBG), which controls circulating oestrogen and testosterone.

As your liver controls the amount of oestrogen circulating in your bloodstream, you need to treat it with respect so it does this job efficiently.

You can help to improve your liver function by making sure that you are taking a good multivitamin and mineral that contains B vitamins and magnesium, as these nutrients help your liver to detoxify oestrogen and render it harmless.

46

Phytoestrogens such as soya and lentils help to stimulate your liver to produce SHBG, which controls excess hormones, and also flaxseeds (linseeds) can stimulate the production of SHBG and aid the removal of excess oestrogens out of your body.[15] Include these foods in your diet and also add artichokes and dandelion greens as they help your liver produce bile, which is needed to break fats down into small molecules so that they can be digested. Onions, leeks and garlic are also beneficial for your liver as they contain sulphur compounds, which are important for efficient liver function. Other vegetables that contain these sulphur compounds are the cruciferous vegetables such as cabbage, cauliflower and broccoli; these help the liver to detoxify efficiently.

The herb milk thistle (*Silybum marianum*) is the herb of choice for boosting liver function; you can take it on its own or combined with other herbs that help with menopausal symptoms such as black cohosh and agnus castus. (The combination I use in the clinic is NHP's Black Cohosh Plus, which contains milk thistle and agnus castus plus dong quai and sage. See www.naturalhealthpractice.com.)

STEP 12: AVOID REFINED SUGAR

This may be the last step in my Twelve-Step Hormone Balancing Diet, but for me as a nutritionist it is one of the most important. Over the 30 years that I have been practising, this is the change in lifestyle that has had the biggest impact on the health and lives of the women that I see. I know this sounds dramatic but all I can say is try it and see.

Throughout the rest of this part of the book, you will see the enormous impact that too much refined sugar and other refined carbohydrates has on your health and that reducing and/or eliminating them is far more important than reducing fat. Sugar is just empty calories and carries no nutritional value.

What effect does sugar have on your health?

The impact of refined sugar on your health is enormous because it creates a domino effect on many organs, glands and systems in your body. Some of the symptoms associated with the effects of sugar are:

- tiredness
- mood swings – irritability, crying spells, aggressive outbursts
- anxiety and tension
- inability to concentrate
- headaches
- dizziness
- palpitations
- forgetfulness
- weight gain – especially around the middle
- lack of sex drive
- high cholesterol
- thyroid problems
- Type 2 diabetes
- feeling more stressed

Many of these symptoms, which you might think are due to a particular stage of the menopause, really have nothing to do with it – they are caused by the effect of refined sugar and refined carbohydrates on your body and your health.

When I talk about refined sugar I mean any sugar that does not naturally occur in that food and has been added as an ingredient. So, for instance, there is fruit sugar in fruit but it is *meant to be there* and is therefore classed as *unrefined*. But if fructose (powdered fruit sugar) has been added to a product then that fructose is *refined*. Sugar in a breakfast cereal has been added by the manufacturers and is classed as *refined*.

HOW MUCH SUGAR DO WE EAT?

We are buying fewer bags of sugar these days, but our sugar consumption in the UK has risen by 31 per cent over the last 20 years to 1¼lb (0.5kg) per person per week.[16] In the US, over the same period of time, the consumption has gone from ½lb (0.2kg) per person per week to nearly 3lb (1.3kg) per person per week. During the late nineteenth century, the average consumption was 5lb (2.2kg) per person per year.

Just what is the problem with refined sugar?

When you eat unrefined carbohydrates, such as oats and brown rice, your body gets a gradual release of glucose into the bloodstream and a certain amount of insulin is released from the pancreas to deal with this gradual rise in blood sugar. But foods and drinks that contain refined sugar cause a rapid and high rise in blood sugar. Your body has to respond to this by producing more insulin from the pancreas to deal with the high level of blood sugar.

The higher your blood sugar goes up, the lower it crashes down afterwards. At the drop (and the drop will also occur if you go longer than three hours without eating) your body will do two things: firstly, it will send you off for a quick sugar fix (like a bar of chocolate) because it needs to lift the blood sugar up again; and, at the same time, it releases the stress hormones adrenaline and cortisol from your adrenal glands to release your own sugar stores to try to correct the low level.

This means you can end up on a perpetual roller-coaster of highs and lows, which will affect your moods, make you feel more anxious and tense because stress hormones are being released, and can make you gain weight, especially around your middle. (For more on this, see chapter 10.)

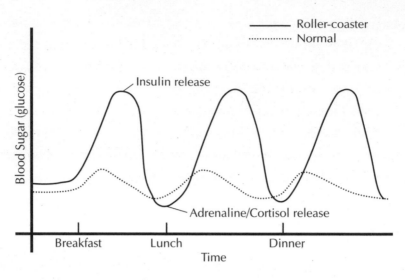

THE BLOOD SUGAR ROLLER-COASTER

With these constant highs and lows, your body will eventually stop responding to insulin, meaning the cells become lazy. Your pancreas may even try to produce more insulin to try and get the cells to respond but the cells have become insulin resistant, resulting in Type 2 diabetes. Insulin-sensitising medications are often given at this stage to try and get the body to respond to insulin again. There can also be a stage when the pancreas doesn't produce enough insulin so a person may need two lots of medication: one to help the pancreas produce more insulin and the insulin sensitiser to help the body to respond to whatever insulin is produced. This is a desperate situation and one that can be avoided.

You *can* prevent Type 2 (middle age onset) diabetes, even if it runs in the family, by changing your diet and eliminating refined sugar in all its forms. Also, many of the symptoms you are suffering that you think are related to the menopause may in fact not be. Change your diet first and you will then see what underlying symptoms are really being caused by the stage of the menopause you are in and not by blood sugar fluctuations.

Sugar in the products you buy

Read the labels on what you buy. Sugar is added not only to the obvious sweet things but also to products such as mayonnaise, tomato ketchup, baked beans and spaghetti sauces. If you look around you will find that there is usually an alternative brand available that does not have sugar added.

If the label says 'no added sugar', check that an artificial sweetener has not been added instead. Sugar comes in many forms and if you see any of these in an ingredient list on a food buy something else:

- fructose (fruit sugar)
- glucose (made from starch and is the same form of carbohydrate that your body uses)
- dextrose (sugar from cornstarch, chemically identical to glucose)
- lactose (milk sugar)
- maltose (made from starch)
- sucrose (common table white or brown sugar, made from sugar cane or beet)
- corn syrup (made from corn, but the effect is the same as sucrose).

Ingredients on a label are always listed in terms of the highest amounts first so manufacturers break down the sugar content into different forms of sugars so it is not listed as the first ingredient. It is currently impossible to ascertain the total amount of added sugar by reading a product's ingredients list or the nutrition information.

The UK Food Standards Agency is aware of this and has published a report entitled 'Investigation of consumer understanding of sugars labelling . . . with specific reference to breakfast cereals'.[17] One comment from the report stated that 'there was great surprise when the stimulus boards showed the red signposts for sugars on the cereals which respondents had previously considered healthy, such as mueslis and bran-type cereals. Indeed there was generally a great deal of shock at high sugar levels across the board on almost all cereals, even though they knew there is "added sugar" in sugary cereals.'

This report highlights how misleading food labelling can be. The hype on the front of the packet may emphasise some of the good things about the food, such as being high in fibre, but omits to show that it is loaded with added sugar. As consumers we should be able to see clearly what is in a product so we can make an informed choice and compare products easily to see which one is healthier. The aim in the EU had been to have a 'traffic light' system of food labels, where red, green and amber symbols would be added to food packs to show if a product had high, medium or low amounts of ingredients that could potentially be harmful. This would have been easy to see on a supermarket shelf and easy to understand. In 2010 this system was rejected by the EU after a campaign by supermarkets and food manu-facturers who were worried that their sales would be affected.

Shockingly, many breakfast cereals can contain more sugar than a doughnut. One popular brand has 11.1g of sugar in a 30g serving (3 teaspoons of sugar per small bowl) while a doughnut has 8.6g of sugar.

Many of the women I see in the clinic are buying low fat or no fat fruit yogurts (even organic ones), but they can contain up to *8 teaspoons of sugar in one pot*. It does not matter if the added sugar is organic or not, the effect on your body is the same.

And what about the so-called 'healthy' probiotic drinks? These often contain sugar, perhaps in the form of glucose-fructose syrup. You would be better off taking a probiotic supplement than swallow-ing this sugar-laden drink.

You may decide to take less sugar in your tea or coffee but it is the hidden added sugar in food products that can be the major culprit in your diet. It has been calculated that we could be taking in up to 46 teaspoons of added sugar in a day in the foods and drinks that we consume (savoury and sweet).[18] Change over to a sugar-free brand of tomato ketchup or spaghetti sauce, swap your sugary jam for a pure fruit version and you will find that you will not taste any difference. Try using a small amount of honey, maple syrup, barley malt, agave nectar or rice syrup if you want a bit of sweetness. You can also use xylitol, which is naturally found in fruits and berries and has a low GI. You can use it in the same way as sugar. Use dried fruit in recipes to add sweetness – I use dessert apples rather than tart cooking apples to make apple crumble and also add sultanas to the apples instead of adding sugar. (See my cookbook *Healthy Eating for the Menopause* (Kyle Cathie) for sweet and savoury recipes all made without added sugar.)

FOOD SUPPLEMENTS

I believe the well-balanced diet is a myth and although I have made suggestions for how to eat healthily, indicating what foods to include and what to avoid, I do think that food supplements are an important addition to our diet. There are a number of reasons for this. One is that food itself does not contain the nutrients it used to. For example, *The Independent Food Commission's Food Magazine* found that, compared to the 1930s, the fruits and vegetables we eat contain an average of 20 per cent fewer minerals (magnesium 24 per cent, calcium 46 per cent, iron 27 per cent and zinc 59 per cent). With regard to meat and dairy, iron in meat has been depleted by 47 per cent, iron in milk by over 60 per cent, calcium loss in cheese by 15 per cent and in Parmesan cheese by 70 per cent.

The problem is that even with our best intentions the soil that our food is grown in has become depleted in vital nutrients from over-farming and the use of pesticides. Also, many fruits and vegetables are flown hundreds of miles and can sit in a warehouse for a period of time before getting to the shelves, creating yet more nutrient depletion. Additionally, if you buy ready-prepared vegetables, such as sliced carrots, they will contain fewer nutrients than if you took the whole carrot home and cut it up just before cooking.

The other factor to take into consideration when thinking about supplements is that during or just before the menopause your body is going through a transition. Giving it extra support with certain key nutrients will help you to go through this phase smoothly.

As well as the here and now, you should also be thinking about prevention for the future. Increasing your intake of nutrients such as calcium, vitamin D, magnesium, zinc, antioxidants and fish oils can make a big difference to the future health of your bones and heart.

In each section of the book, I will discuss the most important supplements to take and why, and explain why they are so essential for your future health.

WHEN FOOD SUPPLEMENTS MIGHT BE USEFUL

Food supplements are important even for women who are eating well but there are certain groups of women who are going to need them even more. Food supplements can be especially helpful in the following cases.

If you don't eat a particularly healthy diet

If you eat fewer than five total servings of fruits and vegetables daily, you may not be getting all of the vitamins and minerals your body needs. Also, if you eat only once or twice a day, you may be limiting the number and variety of foods that you eat.

If you're a vegan

If you're a vegan you may not be getting enough vitamin B12, which is found mainly in animal foods. A good multivitamin and mineral would give you adequate vitamin B12 plus other nutrients.

If you consume fewer than 1,200 calories a day

Low-calorie diets limit the types and amounts of foods you eat and, in turn, the types and amounts of nutrients you take in.

If you have a medical condition that affects how your body absorbs, uses or excretes nutrients

If your diet has limited variety because of food allergies or intolerance to certain foods, for example if you have coeliac disease, food supplements can be especially beneficial.

If you suffer from heavy menstrual bleeding

If you have heavy periods, you may need additional iron to replace the iron depleted by blood loss. Iron deficiency can lead to anaemia, a condition in which blood is low in haemoglobin, the substance that carries oxygen to cell tissues. Symptoms of anaemia can include feeling tired, exhaustion, shortness of breath, dizziness, sore tongue and headaches. If tests suggest that you are iron-deficient, take extra iron. Vitamin C is essential for the body to absorb iron, so for maximum absorption take a vitamin C supplement with your iron supplement on an empty stomach. Avoid taking iron and vitamin C alongside any other supplements you may be taking. Avoid taking iron in the form of ferrous sulphate (also called iron sulphate), which is less easily absorbed by the body. Only 2 to 10 per cent of the iron from this type of iron supplement is actually absorbed by your body, and even then, half is eliminated, causing blackening of your stools and constipation. Ferrous sulphate is classed as an inorganic iron. Organic irons are much more easily absorbed and do not affect the bowels in same way. (If you need help finding organic iron supplements go to www.naturalhealthpractice.com.)

If you smoke

Tobacco decreases the absorption of many vitamins and minerals, including vitamin C, folic acid, magnesium and calcium. But food supplements can't make up for the major health risks caused by smoking. The safest, and of course healthiest, option is to stop smoking.

If you drink alcohol excessively

Long-term excessive alcohol consumption can impair the digestion and absorption of several vitamins and minerals, including the B vitamins (including folic acid), iron, zinc, calcium and magnesium. In addition, you may be substituting alcohol for food, resulting in a diet lacking in essential nutrients. Excessive drinking is defined as more than 14 units a week for women (if you drank more than one large glass of wine a day you would exceed this limit). Taking food supplements can be helpful but they can't make up for the major health risks caused by excessive alcohol consumption, so your first goal should be to reduce the amount you drink.

The most important thing to remember is that supplements are just that – *supplementary* to your diet and not a substitute for a healthy one. Your goal should always be to eat well. Supplements are like a sort of health insurance, not a replacement for eating properly.

HOW TO TAKE SUPPLEMENTS

I recommend that you always have a multivitamin and mineral as the foundation of your supplement programme. That way you have a good range of nutrients and you can simply add on whatever extra you need, depending on your situation. So if a particular recommendation in this book suggests 50mg zinc and there is 25mg in the multivitamin then you only need an extra supplement containing 25mg.

The food you consume contains an array of different nutrients – vitamins, minerals, amino acids, essential fats – and these nutrients work together in many different ways in your body.

Your multivitamin and mineral is an important supplement and should be the best quality you can get because it forms the basis of everything else you take. By choosing a good multivitamin and mineral that is formulated especially for women going through the menopause you receive an excellent healthy base to build upon.

When you eat, your food gives you many different combined nutrients and some of the nutrients enable others to be absorbed. For instance, it is important to take vitamin D with calcium, as vitamin D is responsible for calcium absorption in your digestive system – it transports calcium across the wall of the intestines and helps to move calcium into the bone. If you just took a calcium supplement without any vitamin D your body could struggle to digest and absorb that mineral efficiently. Magnesium is also important because it converts vitamin D into its active form that in turn enables calcium to be absorbed. So you can see how important it is to have combinations of nutrients rather than just taking a few separate ones on their own.

Research was published in 2010 which suggested that taking calcium supplements could increase the risk of heart attacks for women,[19] but what was interesting about this review was that it focused only on those women taking calcium on its own and not combined with either vitamin D or other vitamins and minerals.

You will never get enough vitamin C in a multivitamin and mineral so that always needs to be taken separately, but in conjunction with your multivitamin and mineral. You will need to take Omega 3 fish oils separately because, again, the dose would be too small in a multi.

WHAT YOU SHOULD LOOK FOR IN FOOD SUPPLEMENTS

You get what you pay for when buying supplements so it is worth paying extra for quality because, in my experience, with the cheaper ones either the dosages are not high enough and/or the nutrients are in a form that makes them difficult to absorb. You could be wasting your money because your body cannot use them properly. So what should you look for?

I recommend that you always buy capsules. Your body has to work hard when you swallow a tablet because the nutrients are compressed, with the help of binders, into a hard tablet that your body then needs to break down in order to get at the nutrients. With a capsule, your body only has to melt the capsule in order to get at the nutrients inside. Vegetarian capsules are preferable to those made from bovine gelatine. There are now some excellent fish oil capsules that are made with fish oil gelatine rather than bovine gelatine. Take 1,000mg fish oil per day, with 770mg EPA and 510mg DHA.

The second point is to *read the label*. Don't get seduced by the hype in the large print or a long list of impressive-sounding ingredients. What else has been added to this product? Check for unwanted ingredients that have been added, such as colourings and also either sugar, fructose or artificial sweeteners, especially if is a chewable or fizzy tablet. You want to avoid these!

Look at this example of the ingredients in a bottle of vitamin B6 tablets bought on the high street:

Calcium hydrogen phosphate dihydrate, rice starch, microcrystalline cellulose, pyridoxine hydrochloride (B6), stearic acid, hypromellose, magnesium stearate (vegetable origin), talc, titanium dioxide, glycerol, ferrous oxide red.

These are mainly just fillers and binders (in fact, almost everything except the magnesium stearate and B6). Plus the B6 isn't in an easy-to-absorb form (pyridoxine). Compare this to a vitamin B6 that I use in the clinic which are capsules and contain just:

Pyridoxal-5-phosphate (B6), cellulose, silica, vegetable magnesium stearate.

TIPS FOR CHOOSING FOOD SUPPLEMENTS

- Avoid minerals in the form of oxides, sulphates and carbonates. These inorganic forms are more difficult to absorb, which means that your body has to work harder to get the benefit from them.

- Choose minerals in the form of citrates. For example, calcium citrate as this form of calcium is almost 30 per cent more absorbable than calcium carbonate.[20] With vitamin E choose the form that says d-alpha-tocopherol, as this is the natural version of vitamin E. Dl-alpha-tocopherol is the synthetic version and is not so easily absorbed.

- Choose vitamin B6 as pyridoxal-5-phosphate. This is the active form of B6, which your body can use. If you choose a supplement where the B6 is in the form of pyridoxine (a much cheaper form) your body has to convert it in order to get the benefit.

- Always make sure that the vitamin D is in the form of D3, also called cholecalciferol. There is a cheaper form called D2 (ergo-calciferol) but it is not as beneficial as D3 in correcting deficiencies in your body. In fact, researchers found that D3 is nearly twice as effective.[21]

- With vitamin C, choose the alkaline ascorbate form rather than ascorbic acid, so on the label it will say magnesium ascorbate for instance, which is the alkaline form of vitamin C.

- With fish oils, don't just look at the amount of fish oil, which might say 1,000mg. The most important piece of information is the amount of EPA and DHA that the supplement contains which may be on the back of the label. You are aiming for 770mg EPA and 510mg DHA per day. (See NHP's Omega 3 Plus at www.naturalhealthpractice.com.)

The B6 in these capsules is in the active form (pyridoxal-5-phosphate) that your body actually uses, so your body has to do the least amount of work to absorb it. In the pyridoxine form in the tablets your body has to convert the pyridoxine to pyridoxal-5-phosphate to absorb it and if it does not do that successfully, you are wasting your money.

(To see a listing of all the different supplement companies I have chosen to use in the clinic including BioCare, Solgar, Lambert's, Nutri and the Natural Health Practice go to www.naturalhealthpractice.com. I have also formulated some specific supplements for the Natural Health Practice because I couldn't find the right combinations or quality I needed in the clinic – see Useful resources, page 284.)

HERBS

Herbs can be very powerful tools when you are going through the menopause and as I look at the different stages in this book I will highlight the herbs that are the most useful.

Herbal medicine is a traditional and ancient form of medicine and many of the drugs we use today have been derived from it. An example is aspirin (acetylsalicylic acid), which is derived from the bark of the white willow tree. As far back as Hippocrates, around 400BC, it was noted that powder made from the bark of the white willow tree helped with pain relief and headaches. In 1829, a compound named salicin was found to be the active ingredient in willow. This compound was an impure form and a few years later scientists split the salicin and converted it into salicylic acid. This salicylic acid was hard on the stomach, however, so scientists found a way of buffering it to cushion its effect. The end result was acetylsalicylic acid or aspirin as we know it.

I have gone into some detail about how aspirin was formulated from the white willow bark because it is so relevant today. White willow is still used as a herbal remedy; its effects may be slower than aspirin but they last longer, and what is important is that it does not have the same side effects that aspirin can have (including bleeding in the stomach or gut). When we take a herbal remedy in its whole form (in this case the bark of the willow), rather than just the active ingredient, nature provides the plant with buffering substances that counteract the side effects.

Although salicin is thought to be the active ingredient, research is now showing that other compounds in the willow bark also have the ability to reduce fever, decrease inflammation and boost the immune system. So it may be that a number of compounds together in willow combine to create a beneficial effect and that scientists have actually only picked up on one.

USING HERBS

I recommend that when you use herbs you should opt for the whole part of that herb (whether it is the leaf or root) and avoid standardised extracts. If you see the words 'standardised extract' on the label this means that the active ingredient in that herbal remedy is at a guaranteed dose. The implication therefore is that the manufacturer knows precisely what the active ingredient is and that it is 'better' to have it in that strength.

One good example of this is St John's wort. It was believed that the active ingredient that helped with depression was hypericin. Standardised hypericin extracts of St John's wort became available to buy but it has been suggested that hypericin plays only a small part in the action of this powerful herb and that other compounds are also important. Having a higher strength of hypericin compared to the other compounds (which would not occur naturally) has caused the contraindications with certain medications. A few years back a herb called kava kava was removed from the shelves because of concerns over liver problems but the products reported were all standardised extracts, not whole herbs.

When we play around with nature, there are usually consequences, and as with food, we should take herbs in their whole state where possible without them being too refined or processed. The same rule applies to herbs as it does to supplements: always buy the best quality herbs you can and organic where possible. You can either take them in tincture form (where they have been preserved with alcohol) or in capsules (vegetarian preferably) filled with the dried herb. Avoid herbs that come in tablet form as it is likely that other ingredients that may not be desirable will have been added and the tablets will also be more difficult to absorb. Some herbal remedies such as Black Cohosh Plus I have formulated for use in my clinic for the Natural Health Practice because I wanted certain combinations of organic whole herbs that I could not find on the market (see www.naturalhealthpractice.com).

CHAPTER 3

EXERCISE – FOR TODAY AND TOMORROW

You are no doubt aware how important exercise is for a healthy heart, but you may not realise how far the benefits of exercise extend to your general health, especially through the menopause and beyond.

As human beings we are meant to be active. Just a generation ago the norm was to do frequent but low level physical activity on a day-to-day basis; for example, I can remember my mother washing, scrubbing and wringing out clothes by hand. Every day she would walk to the shops and carry back the shopping, and my father would walk to work. There were very few labour-saving devices back then.

Today, the norm is to sit down all day, use the lift or the escalator, then drive the car to the gym for 30 minutes or more of intense exercise. For most people, low-level physical activity is now not part of everyday life, which means we have to consciously take time out to do it by joining a gym or going to an exercise class.

I recommend you not only set aside specific time in which to exercise, but that you also try to 'sneak in' bits of exercise whenever you can – even a 10-minute walk at lunchtime is worth while. It may only seem a small thing but it does matter that you walk up the stairs rather than taking the lift, which increases the risk of both heart disease and diabetes.[1] An interesting study in 2007 looked at a group of women over a period of six and a half years. The researchers found that all types of exercise cut the risk of breast cancer but the strongest link was with housework.[2] Housework is an activity that is done frequently and consistently and seems to give more benefit than short bursts of activity. It is estimated that we burn over 50,000 calories a year doing household chores, which equates to about 57 hours of steady running. Vacuuming uses up over 6,000 calories a year, and dusting and polishing just over 2,000. Ironing and washing-up are also pretty good calorie burners at over 2,500 each.

WHY IS EXERCISE SO IMPORTANT AS YOU GO THROUGH THE MENOPAUSE?

Our two main health risks past the menopause are heart disease and osteoporosis so no matter what stage of the menopause you are at, you must make the effort to keep fit and healthy in order to help prevent them. Exercise, alongside a healthy diet, can help you do that.

As well as the heart and bone benefits, physical activity can help lift your mood, as it releases endorphins, brain chemicals which alleviate depression, release stress and give you a sense of wellbeing. It can also help reduce high blood pressure, boost your immune function, alleviate constipation and prevent Type 2 diabetes. Moreover, as mentioned above, it can cut your risk of breast cancer.

EXERCISE AND HEART DISEASE

When you exercise you are strengthening both your heart and your lungs. The American Heart Association (www.heart.org) states that as a woman you are twice as likely to get heart disease if you are inactive. Lack of physical activity has been strongly linked to heart disease, the biggest killer for women, so it is crucial for us to build exercise into our daily routine.[3]

Exercise also helps to lower total cholesterol, increase HDL 'good' cholesterol and lower LDL 'bad' cholesterol.[4] Heart disease and other degenerative conditions such as arthritis are connected with inflammation and it has been shown that exercise can help to control chronic inflammation.[5]

A study presented at the European Society of Cardiology in Germany in 2008 showed that by banning the use of escalators and lifts at work, the hospital workers who took part in the study had a 15 per cent cut in the risk of dying prematurely. After 12 weeks, the workers had a 2.3 per cent drop in blood pressure, 3.9 per cent in LDL and a reduction in waist circumference and body fat levels. So while these measures might sound draconian, 'sneaking in' exercise as you go about your day can make a huge difference to your health.

EXERCISE AND DIABETES
With 15 per cent of the UK population on the way to developing Type 2 diabetes, it is so important that you do everything you can to avoid this illness. Taking action is even more important if you have a strong family history of this disease. The good news is that a study in the *British Medical Journal* has shown that regular exercise, along with a healthy diet, is as effective as taking prescription diabetic medication. Making healthy lifestyle changes halved the risk of developing Type 2 diabetes.[6]

EXERCISE AND IMMUNE FUNCTION
In case you need more reasons to exercise, it can help boost your immune function.[7] It can help ward off colds and in one study women who walked just 30 minutes a day had half the number of colds of women who were not physically active.[8]

EXERCISE AND ANTI-AGEING
Making regular exercise part of your weekly routine will keep you looking and feeling younger for longer. A study looking at over 20,000

twins found that in the twin who regularly exercised the telomeres (a region of DNA that protects chromosomes from damage and shortens as we age) were longer, indicating that they were ageing more slowly than their twin who was less active.[9]

EXERCISE AND DETOXIFICATION

Your lymphatic system plays an important part in detoxification and immune function. Lymph is a watery yellowish fluid, which accumulates bacteria and waste to be filtered out through the lymphatic system. Unlike your heart, your lymphatic system doesn't have a pump action and relies on your body's musculature movement (the lungs and muscles) to shift lymph around your body, which is another reason why regular exercise is so crucial.

As well as exercise in general, specific activities such as jumping on a rebounder (mini-trampoline) and moving your body as in dancing are beneficial. This can help with water retention and improving the circulation.

EXERCISE AND CANCER

As mentioned at the beginning of this chapter, many studies have shown that taking regular exercise reduces the risk of breast cancer. In fact, walking for just half-an-hour a day has been shown to halve the risk of developing breast cancer.[10]

As well as helping to prevent breast cancer, thirty minutes of exercise a day can also help to lower the risk of bowel cancer by up to a quarter. Bowel cancer is one of the most common cancers and exercise provides beneficial preventive effects independent of obesity, smoking and diet.[11]

The overarching message from all the research, however, is that it is the *total amount* of exercise that is important rather than the type or the intensity.

EXERCISE TIPS

START GENTLY

If you have not been exercising regularly, take things gently at first and begin by walking for 10 minutes, then increasing it until you are walking for 30 minutes at a brisk pace.

GET A PEDOMETER

It is easy to overestimate how active we really are and in actual fact many of us end up sitting or lying down for up to 20 hours a day. Try investing in a pedometer to count how many steps you take on a daily basis. The recommendation is to aim for 10,000 steps each day.

RING THE CHANGES

If you are bored with your exercise routine and you are doing the same thing every week, then it is a good idea to make changes. Your body is very clever at adapting your muscles to whatever exercise you are doing, meaning it will make less of an impact. It is therefore much better to vary the physical activity you do as it will then target different muscle groups and give your body more of a challenge.

INCREASE THE INTENSITY

You could build up the intensity of your workout by picking up the pace for one to three minutes, then returning to your normal pace for three to five minutes. Repeat this cycle throughout your workout as it will help you burn more fat.

EXERCISE FIRST THING

If you can, try to exercise first thing in the morning as this will kick-start your metabolism and help you to burn fat stores all day. If you aren't used to morning exercise make sure you have a light snack such as a piece of fruit and a cracker before you begin; then have your breakfast after your workout and include more protein such as an egg. The protein helps feed your muscles and builds them up after you have used them in the exercise.

INCLUDE WEIGHT TRAINING

Are you doing enough weight training? Muscles require more energy to function than fat does, so if you increase your muscle mass you'll raise the speed at which you burn calories and, consequently, shed fat. Often women try to lose weight by cutting calories and only doing aerobic exercise such as walking, but this means you will lose muscle along with fat. The secret is to maximise fat loss while maintaining muscle tone. Keep doing aerobic activity but start weight training or muscle toning exercises for a slimmer, firmer body. If you do training with weights make sure you have a rest day in between sessions.

FIND AN EXERCISE PARTNER

Making a commitment to exercise with a friend makes it harder to miss a few days, because you know your friend is relying on you to keep them motivated and it is harder to let them down.

BE PREPARED

If you work all day, you might find it easier to exercise first thing in the morning; it just means getting ready the night before so that you take your work clothes to the gym. If you prefer to exercise in the evening, the best approach is to go straight from work. It is all too easy to go home, thinking you will then go to the gym a bit later and find yourself putting it off.

LISTEN TO MUSIC

According to a recent study, fast-paced music has been shown to inspire people to run faster on a treadmill than people who have no music to listen to. So, if you're having trouble getting motivated choose an album of upbeat music that really fires you up and play it both when you work out and when you are getting ready to work out.[12]

DESKERCISE: EXERCISES TO DO AT YOUR DESK

If your job is desk bound there are plenty of things you can do to keep fit and toned. As well as making sure you get up and have a stretch or a short walk every half-an-hour or so try some of the following exercises today:

1. **Calf stretch:** Remove your shoes and place your feet flat on the floor with your knees slightly apart. Bring your toes up towards the front of your legs while keeping your heels on the floor. This will help iron kinks out of your calves.

2. **60-second aerobics:** While seated, pump both arms over your head for 30 seconds, then rapidly tap your feet on the floor, football-drill style, for 30 seconds. Repeat three to five times.

3. **Body lift.** Place your hands on the arms of your chair and lift yourself up slightly. Repeat.

4. **Buttock squeeze:** Tighten and squeeze your buttocks, hold for 5 to 10 seconds, and release. Repeat six to eight times. Really concentrate on the 'squeeze' for maximum results.

5. **Straight and narrow:** Sit up straight in your chair. Take note of how you sit throughout the day. If you're slumping a lot, try to practise correcting your posture. Good posture makes you look thinner.

6. **Arch:** While sitting up arrow straight, bring your lower tummy forward until you feel your back arch. Next, reverse the motion. This will help relieve back pressure.

SHORT OF TIME?

Many women tell me that they can't exercise because they don't have enough time and just trying to fit something else into their busy lives makes them feel more stressed. I do understand, but having some form of physical activity in the day should be as important as cleaning your teeth and you have to fit in the time to do that. Could you spare 12 minutes in a day? Well, if you can, then there is an easy solution. In the 1950s an exercise programme was designed for Canadian pilots whose space and time was limited. It was called 5BX (Five Basic Exercises) and became a worldwide fitness phenomenon as it was very popular with office workers and the book sold 23 million copies. The five exercises are stretches, sit-ups, back arches and press-ups followed by a short aerobic workout. You can find details of it on the website www.gettingfitagain.com.

EASY EXERCISES FOR INCREASING MUSCLE MASS

SQUATS

This is an easy exercise you can do at home, even in front of the television, which helps to build muscles.

Stand with your back straight, chest lifted and abdominals in. Tilt your pelvis forward. Breathe in as you bend from your knees and hips and slowly squat down. Keep your weight over your ankles. Look forward. As you squat, extend your arms straight in front of you at or below shoulder height. Keep your back flat, chest lifted and knees in line with your feet. Don't allow the squat to go beyond seat height. Keep your thighs parallel to the floor. Breathe out as you slowly stand

VIBRATING PLATES

Vibrating plates have recently become popular in many gyms and have been promoted as a useful piece of exercise equipment for preventing and even reversing osteoporosis.

There are basically two different ways that the plates move and it is this difference that I think is very important. Some of these pieces of equipment have plates that vibrate in three planes including side to side in a horizontal motion (whole body vibrators) and others, which only vibrate up and down.

I have concerns about the machines that vibrate the whole body. They deliver a shaking motion, which can be in three directions at the same time (side to side, front to back, and up and down). My concern is that this vibrating effect and the range of motion can be too extreme for some people, especially the elderly, but also for those whose bones may have less than optimum bone density. It seems that this type of machine is more appropriate for improving muscle strength as they cause fast and short contractions in muscle and tendons.

I think the machines that offer only a vertical motion have much more to offer with regard to the prevention and treatment of osteoporosis. They provide a low level of vibration in an up and down motion that causes the muscle fibres to twitch. When you think of the exercises recommended for improving bone density, such as walking and jogging, the emphasis is on having an impact through a vertical motion with the ground. As I see it, the vertical motion machines are imitating those exercises but just in a more concentrated way.

With either type of machine, there is not much scientific evidence regarding their effects on bone health and given a choice I would have to recommend the vertical motion rather than the whole body vibrators, as these replicate our own natural movements when we exercise.

up. Lead with your shoulders and keep your back flat and heels on the floor. Try to complete one set of 12 to 15 repetitions. Once you get the hang of it, try increasing to 20 reps and then increase the number of sets you complete.

LUNGES

Another exercise you can do at home that improves your muscle mass. Stand with feet shoulder-width apart and take a big step forward with your right leg, making sure your knee stops above your ankle and doesn't bend more than 90 degrees. Foot planted, shift your weight onto your right leg and bring your left foot beside the right. Lead with alternate legs (10 to 12 reps each leg).

CHAPTER 4

ANTI-AGEING AND HOW TO SLOW DOWN THE CLOCK

'As you get older three things happen.
The first is your memory goes, and I can't
remember the other two' – Norman Wisdom

No matter what age you are, most women want to age as slowly as possible. And for me that means slowing down the age process from the inside and the outside. The earlier you can start following the recommendations in this chapter and the dietary advice in chapter 2 the better. The more you can do before the change in hormones at the menopause the easier the transition and the slower the ageing process. But it is never too late. Your body is really adaptable and given the right diet and nutrients, these can make a big impact on not only your health but also how fast you age, regardless of when you start.

In my view, it is really important to know what you can do to control the ageing process from inside your body as this will not only help you to look and feel good but it can also help to safeguard your long-term health. As well as wanting to slow down the ageing process, everyone wants to live a long and healthy life. The two go hand in hand because what you do to slow down the clock will help to give you quantity of years but with the benefit of quality of life to go with it. With the prospect of living 30 to 50 years past the menopause, you want to live those years not only looking and feeling good for your age but also with the energy and health to carry on being independent and doing the things you want to do, with a sharp mind and healthy body.

There are some simple things that you can put into place now that will slow down the clock, so although you will of course grow older you will not age as fast.

No matter what age you are, you can still take steps to slow down the clock. Obviously the younger you start the more impact you can have on how you look and feel, but it is never too late to start leading

HOW LONG DOES IT TAKE FOR DIFFERENT PARTS OF YOUR BODY TO REGENERATE?

- **Bones:** It takes about 10 years to replace your skeleton, which is constantly renewing itself. Your entire skeleton is made up of new bone that was not there 10 years before. But as we get older the process of renewal can take longer.
- **Hair:** An individual hair is replaced after six years.
- **Intestines:** The villi in the intestines are replaced every two to three days.
- **Eyes:** The only part of the eye that can be renewed is the cornea.
- **Liver:** Liver cells are replaced every five months.
- **Brain:** There are only two parts of the brain that regenerate, namely the area governing the sense of smell and the hippocampus, the area for learning.
- **Skin:** Regenerates every two to four weeks but as we age there are changes in the skin as collagen and elasticity are lost.

an 'anti-ageing' lifestyle. Your body regenerates itself all the time, with different cells replacing themselves at differing rates. So you have the potential to start creating healthy cells right now!

WHAT MAKES US AGE?

There are a number of theories about what causes ageing, but no definitive answer. I believe that a combination of factors make us age, not just one factor, so I will now look at the common issues that are known to accelerate ageing and give you natural solutions to combat them.

1. FREE RADICALS

We generate free radicals through the natural process of living and breathing but we also inhale, absorb and digest them. Free radicals are molecules that come from environmental pollutants, radiation, pesticides, preservatives, cigarettes and car fumes.

Free radical damage has been linked to premature ageing and many of the illnesses that are connected to us getting older, including cancer, heart disease and Alzheimer's disease. And it also plays a significant role in the ageing process of your skin.

Free radicals can affect your skin by damaging the collagen, which would normally give skin its elasticity and softness. Over time free radical damage can make your skin harder and drier, resulting in wrinkles.

The only thing that neutralises free radicals is a group of nutrients known as antioxidants of which the most potent are the powerful natural antioxidants, namely vitamins A, C, E and flavonoids found in fruits and vegetables. When antioxidants are eaten or applied to the skin they help to neutralise free radicals and prevent tissue damage. The message is simple: the more fruit and vegetables you eat the more you reduce your risk of ageing faster, both inside and out.

2. BLOOD SUGAR PROBLEMS

Fluctuating blood sugar levels that cause highs of glucose and insulin make you age faster. This is explained by the Glycation Theory of Ageing, which was introduced in the 1980s, and describes when glucose (sugar) gets out of control. Glycation is the process that changes your body's protein structures (such as your skin, hair, blood vessels and organs) into substances called, appropriately, AGEs (Advanced Glycation End Products).

Your body is 60 per cent protein and when these proteins react with excess sugar from what you eat, they end up causing cells to lose their elasticity; they become hardened and can stop functioning properly. It is the same process that occurs when we cook food and the food ends up becoming brown. When we heat up the top of a crème brûlée, a combination of the proteins from milk together with sugar cause it to end up with a brown hard crust on the top. If you have excess sugar consumption, the same 'browning' effect is going on inside and outside your body causing higher levels of glucose.

This reaction of glucose and proteins damages your cells inside and outside your body and makes you age faster. Scientists have done studies on animals showing that just giving them a small amount of glucose, reduces their life span by 20 per cent.[1]

These AGEs can cause changes in your skin making it less elastic and creating more wrinkles than is appropriate for your age. Also that same hardening effect will be going on inside your body without you being able to see it. This can increase the risk of heart disease (hardening of the arteries), eye problems (like cataracts) and nerve damage (where circulation and feeling deteriorates). These are the exact same complications that diabetics can suffer from because of poorly or uncontrolled glucose.

Changing your cooking techniques can help reduce AGEs; reduce temperatures and cook with water (boil, poach or steam) most of the time instead of dry baking, barbecuing or grilling. Water prevents sugars from binding to protein molecules, so helps reduce the formation of AGEs.

Follow my recommendations on page 47 to get your blood sugar under control and bear in mind that by reducing or eliminating the amount of added sugar in your diet (in cakes, sweets or biscuits) and also reducing refined carbohydrates such as white flour, you can not only extend your life span but also help yourself to stay looking and feeling younger for longer.

3. ENVIRONMENTAL TOXINS

Every day your body is exposed to a sea of environmental toxins such as pesticides, industrial chemicals, car fumes, cigarette smoke and additives and preservatives in processed or refined food. When exposure to these toxins becomes overwhelming the toxins accumulate in your body, damaging cells and contributing to wrinkles and saggy skin. The best way to reduce your risk of wrinkles is to eat a diet that is as fresh, healthy (preferably organic) and rich in whole foods as possible, and to avoid unnecessary exposure to environmental toxins.

4. INFLAMMATION

Another cause of ageing and wrinkles is inflammation. Inflammation can be triggered by stress because at the same time adrenaline is released (as a result of stressors), cortisol is also produced and this hormone produces inflammatory substances called cytokines. Cytokines can calm or stimulate the immune system; they can also cause cells to multiply and divide. Inflammation is also triggered when your cells undergo attack from free radicals. Substances are activated that cause your cells to produce inflammatory agents and as a result further chemicals are produced, which digest available collagen; collagen is what keeps your skin looking fresh and young, so when your skin is under free radical attack it has no defence system in place. If you have fat around the middle of your body, you will produce more of these inflammatory cytokines.

Omega 3 fatty acids (see page 27) help to control inflammation because they produce anti-inflammatory prostaglandins. On the other hand, the Omega 6 fatty acids can produce more of the substances that increase inflammation. Research has shown that people who have diets high in Omega 6 and low in Omega 3 fatty acids produce more inflammation, which is linked to a number of degenerative 'old age' diseases including heart disease and Alzheimer's.[2] Also DHA, which is the major Omega 3 fatty acid in the brain, seems to have the most protective effect against Alzheimer's by preventing plaque forming in the brain.[3,4]

5. STRESS

When you are under long-term stress, whether that stress is physical, emotional, psychological or environmental, your body produces increased levels of cortisol, which can age your body and skin faster. Research has shown that women with the highest stress levels prematurely age by an extra 10 years compared to less stressed women.[5] The stress hormone cortisol also increases free radical damage as well as reducing the antioxidant enzymes that would normally protect your cells from damage.

Vitamin C is important for the manufacture of collagen but it is used up by stress and this too can lead to changes in the skin.

Try and minimise stress by making time for yourself each day. Take 30 minutes to go for a walk in the fresh air, meditate or relax in a bath with soothing essential oils like lavender, chamomile or jasmine. And make sure that you have enough quality sleep each night; this is very important.

6. NOT GETTING ENOUGH SLEEP

During sleep your body repairs its cells and recharges its batteries. One of the hormones released by the pineal gland while you sleep is melatonin, which helps to prevent free radical attack. Your skin and body are under free radical attack every day so every night you need to protect it with a good night's sleep. Melatonin is thought to slow down the ageing process[6] and used to be available in health food shops in the UK and still is in the US, but I do not recommend it. It is a hormone, not a food supplement, and should therefore be prescribed by a medical expert. Rather than resort to such measures, it is much better to improve the quality and quantity of your sleep so that your body produces the correct amount of melatonin required rather than trying to judge how much and when you need it and adding it to your body in an artificial form.

Sleep experts believe that the most important time for skin repair is between 10 p.m. and midnight, so try to get to bed early and aim to eat your evening meal before 8 p.m. so that your body is not digesting when it should be resting.

Lack of sleep is in itself stressful for your body and you can end up producing more of the stress hormones, adrenaline and cortisol, which will also age you.

There is more detail about sleep on page 90.

7. TOO MUCH SUN

The sun's rays can damage the DNA in skin cells and it is thought that the great majority of visible signs of skin ageing in many women, such as wrinkles, age spots (sometimes called liver spots) and sagging skin may be caused by over-exposure to the sun. And even though darker or olive skin may not burn easily, a suntan is basically evidence of injury to the epidermis, the top layer of skin.

Prevention is the best way to reduce the risk of sun damage. Using a sunscreen with more natural ingredients, especially on the face and hands, is important, as is avoiding excessive exposure to the sun. (For more on natural sunscreens go to www.naturalhealthpractice.com.)

8. NOT ENOUGH SUN

You do have to be careful of damage to your skin from sun exposure but ironically you will also age faster if you do not have *enough* sun. Your body manufactures vitamin D through your skin when exposed to the sun. However, it can't do this if you are covered in sunscreen.

As with anything in nature, you don't want too much of something but you also don't want too little. Australia, having for many years promoted messages of staying out of the sun and always using sunscreen, is now recording vitamin D deficiencies in one out of four people.[7]

Over the last few years, our knowledge of the benefits of vitamin D in all areas of our health has greatly increased. I will cover these benefits as they come up in the different sections of the book, but to give an idea of their significance they include prevention of cancer, especially breast cancer, heart disease, Type 2 diabetes and osteoporosis. And one of the main benefits is that vitamin D can slow down the ageing process.

One of the theories of ageing relates to DNA structures called telomeres (mentioned on page 66). These are the protective caps at the end of chromosomes – rather like the hard ends on shoelaces. They get shorter as we get older and scientists have been trying to find ways of stopping this shortening process.

Scientists have found that people with higher vitamin D levels have longer telomere length and were quoted as saying that this 'underscores the potentially beneficial effects of this hormone on ageing and age-related diseases'.[8] Vitamin D can help to control inflammation and it is known that inflammation causes the telomeres to shorten, which is another reason why vitamin D can help slow down the clock.

My recommendation would be to go out in the sun for at least 15 minutes a day (avoiding the hottest part of the day in summer, which is midday to 3 p.m.) without sunscreen and without make-up or moisturiser as most cosmetics now have in-built sun protection factors that will interfere with your body's production of vitamin D. If you have avoided the sun previously or are worried you might be deficient in vitamin D, it is better to have a simple blood test to check your level and then supplement with vitamin D as appropriate (see Useful Resources page 283 if you can't get a vitamin D deficiency test).

9. NOT ENOUGH EXERCISE

We all know that exercise is important for general health. It is good for heart health, depression, constipation, bone health, weight control and much more. But an added benefit is that studies at the US National Institute on Aging have shown that regular walking can seriously slow the ageing process (have a look at www.niapublications.org/tipsheets/pdf/Whats_Your_Aging_IQ.pdf). Just shorten and quicken your pace, swing your arms and do it a lot.

10. EATING TOO MUCH

Over the years research has shown that calorie restriction definitely slows the ageing process and increases life span. Although the emphasis with this type of diet is reducing the intake of calories the aim is also to make the diet nutrient-rich, so that the person is not malnourished.

It has been known for over 80 years that if the daily calories given to mice are reduced by half they live up to 30 per cent longer. Increased life span has also been shown in fish, dogs and yeasts by reducing calories.

In humans it has been calculated that we would have to reduce our calories by 25 to 30 per cent to achieve the same effect. And even though the research on animals has been around for eight decades it is still not clear why calorie restriction has this effect.

Some researchers think that certain genes are activated to help fight disease if the body perceives there is a famine situation, so therefore the body is stronger. Other research suggests that it works by decreasing insulin and therefore stops the AGEs as mentioned above (see page 76).

The first study on humans on a restricted diet in 2006 showed reduced signs of ageing. The men and women on the diet had reduced fasting insulin levels, lowered signs of inflammation and also the rate at which their DNA decayed also slowed, reducing their risk of cancer.[9]

This would not be an easy dietary regime to follow and one I would not recommend as trying to pack all the necessary nutrients into a smaller amount of calories could take over your life. What we can take from this knowledge, however, is not to overeat and you can do this by putting less on your plate. Simple tricks such as using smaller plates can make a big difference as your brain can be tricked into thinking you are full when it sees an empty plate.

Also, take your time when you eat; the first part of digestion happens in your mouth so chew slowly and properly and your food will be digested better. Your brain takes 20 minutes to register that you are full so by eating fast you risk eating more than necessary before your brain tells you you have had enough. By eating more slowly you will have consumed less food and still be satisfied.

PLAN OF ACTION

In order to hold back the years, you need to carefully consider the following points: put into place a good exercise programme, make sure you get enough sleep (see page 90), look at controlling stress (see page 78), get some sunshine and, one of the most important ones, get your blood sugar under control.

There are also two groups of foods that are especially important for controlling the ageing process: Omega 3 essential fatty acids because they control inflammation; and also fruit and vegetables because they supply you with good levels of antioxidants. With regard to Omega 3 essential fatty acids, you should aim to increase your

FOOD	ORAC SCORE PER 100G*
Prunes	5,770
Raisins	2,830
Blueberries	2,400
Blackberries	2,036
Kale	1,770
Strawberries	1,540
Raspberries	1,220
Brussels sprouts	980
Plums	949
Alfalfa sprouts	930
Broccoli florets	890
Beet (beetroot)	840
Oranges	750
Red peppers	710
Red grapes	739
Cherries	670

* Remember, the ORAC score is a measure of the protective value of these foods.

consumption of oily fish (such as mackerel, sardines, pilchards and tuna) and also flaxseeds (linseeds), eggs and soya. With regard to antioxidants, I want to discuss these foods in a bit more detail because this is an exciting area of research and we can learn a lot from the scientific literature available.

Scientists at the US Department of Agriculture have developed a rating scale that measures the antioxidant content of various foods. The scale is called ORAC (oxygen radical absorbance capacity). There are some 'super foods' that contain 20 times the antioxidant power compared to other foods. The aim is to eat 3,000 ORAC units a day and to get them by eating a mixture of different foods. Variety is the key because the scientists who developed the ORAC scale said that combinations of nutrients in foods might have a greater protective effect than each nutrient alone. This is because it's estimated that there are more than 4,000 compounds in foods that act as antioxidants so having a variety of these compounds is going to be better than focusing on one type of antioxidant. Clearly, a handful of prunes provides good protection, but don't think that simply eating a handful of prunes every day will protect you – it's the variety of health-giving foods that's important.

TOP 10 ANTI-AGEING NUTRIENTS

These are the top 10 most important anti-ageing nutrient supplements and their recommended doses.

1. Vitamin C

Vitamin C is a powerful antioxidant, which helps to slow the ageing process. According to the Center for Disease Control and Prevention in the US, people with diabetes have up to 30 per cent lower concentrations of vitamin C, so good vitamin C intakes might aid in the prevention of diabetes.

Vitamin C also helps to reduce cholesterol and lower blood pressure, high levels of which are risk factors for heart disease.

Dose: 500mg twice a day, best as ascorbate (rather than ascorbic acid).

2. Vitamin E

Vitamin E is a fat-soluble antioxidant (meaning it is stored for longer in the liver and fatty tissues) and plays an important role in combating the effects of free radicals, which are linked to premature ageing. Not only does it help to mop up free radicals, it also helps to control glucose, which in turn causes free radical damage to cells. Vitamin E helps to control inflammation and has been shown to help reduce the risk of heart disease and strokes, as it helps to prevent blood clotting abnormally. A study at Cambridge University showed that using 400–800ius of vitamin E a day helped reduce the risk of a heart attack by 75 per cent. It is thought that vitamin E prevents the 'bad' LDL cholesterol from oxidising (or going off) in the blood.

Dose: 400–600ius per day, best as the natural form d-alpha-tocopherol rather than the synthetic dl-alpha-tocopherol.

3. Selenium

Selenium is a powerful antioxidant that helps to protect your body from the highly reactive chemical fragments, free radicals. As we get older, our levels of selenium decline. A number of studies have shown a link between selenium deficiency and cancer and also heart disease. Selenium is an essential mineral for making the enzyme glutathione peroxidase, one of the most important enzymes for neutralising free radicals.

Dose: 100–200μg per day.

4. Alpha-lipoic acid

Alpha-lipoic acid is a powerful antioxidant that is made by the body and its role is to release energy by burning glucose. Keeping glucose under control is crucial as otherwise it speeds up damage to cells and, over time, reactions can occur that cause membranes and blood vessels to thicken and can harden arteries. Over time, blood vessels will lose their elasticity and skin can become wrinkled – all signs of ageing. Alpha-lipoic acid also helps support healthy liver function.

Dose: 100mg per day.

5. Acetyl L-carnitine

The amino acid acetyl L-carnitine has been shown to help with age-related mental decline. It is thought that it increases the brain receptors that would normally deteriorate with age so is helpful for reducing the risk of memory loss, dementia, Alzheimer's and depression. Acetyl

L-carnitine works with co-enzyme Q10 and alpha-lipoic acid to maintain the function of the mitochondria, the power houses of your cells, which provide the energy for your cells to function and survive. As the mitochondria function declines, degenerative disease is inevitable and energy production also decreases.

Dose: 250–500mg per day.

6. Co-enzyme Q10

This vitamin-like substance is contained in nearly every cell of the body. It is important for energy production and normal carbohydrate metabolism (the way the body breaks down the carbohydrates that are eaten in order to turn them into energy). We can become deficient in Q10 as we get older, which can result in depleted energy levels.

Co-enzyme Q10 also has a role in controlling blood sugar levels and helps to lower glucose and insulin. In one randomised double blind trial patients with high blood pressure and taking blood pressure medication, were given co-enzyme Q10.[10] Those taking co-enzyme Q10 had lower blood pressure and increased levels of HDL ('good' cholesterol). Their levels of antioxidant vitamins A, C, E and beta-carotene also increased.

Dose: 25–50mg per day.

7. Omega 3

Omega 3 essential fatty acids are crucial for the correct functioning of cell membranes, which are made up of 60 per cent fat. They help the membranes to be more fluid and flexible, which is important not only for brain function but also heart health and fat burning. Cells and arteries tend to get harder with age, so anything that can slow this down is helpful. The Omega 3 oils also help to lower cholesterol and reduce inflammation, which is connected to ageing.

Dose: 1,000mg per day with 770mg EPA and 510mg DHA.

8. Green tea extract.

Green tea (*Camellia sinensis*) contains polyphenols, which have been found to have anti-cancer properties and also help reduce cholesterol and increase HDL 'good' cholesterol. Polyphenols have also been studied for their effect on weight reduction and loss of body fat, even when the diet remains the same.[11] One of the categories of the polyphenols, catechins, has been shown to inhibit growth of cancer cells by inducing cell death (apoptosis).

Dose: 50mg per day.

9. B vitamins including folic acid

The B vitamins are known as the 'anti-stress' vitamins, and it is well known that stress makes us age faster. Folic acid is also one of the important B vitamins, which, along with vitamins B6 and B12, helps to control a toxic substance called homocysteine that under normal circumstances is detoxified (broken down and excreted) by the body. High levels of homocysteine have been linked to heart disease, Alzheimer's and osteoporosis – diseases associated with getting older.

Dose: B1, B2, B3, B5, B6 – 25mg per day; B12 – 25µg per day; folic acid at least 400µg per day.

10. Ginkgo biloba

Ginkgo biloba is a herb that is useful not only for improving and maintaining memory function but also blood circulation. It is believed to help memory and concentration by stimulating blood flow to the brain by dilating blood vessels and preventing clotting. It also functions as a powerful antioxidant and therefore prevents free radical damage. So this is an important herb for preventing dementia, Alzheimer's and circulatory problems that could come with age.

Dose: 100–150mg per day.

For a good combination of these anti-ageing nutrients see Nutri Plus at www.naturalhealthpractice.com.)

BE WARY OF DHEA

DHEA (dehydroepiandrosterone) is touted as the anti-ageing hormone. It is produced by the body but declines as we get older. It is said to prevent cancer, heart disease and Alzheimer's, but is surrounded by a lot of hype. It is available on the internet but it can come with a price. DHEA is a steroid hormone; it is not a food or a vitamin or mineral supplement. The body easily converts DHEA into oestrogen and testosterone so must be used with extreme caution in people with hormonal cancers. Other noted side effects are palpitations, excess growth of body hair and also hair loss (male pattern baldness).

TOP 10 ANTI-AGEING FOODS

1. Berries
All the berries have good amounts of antioxidants. Eat a variety to get the different kinds of antioxidants.

2. Oily fish (mackerel, herring, pilchards, tuna etc.)
Contain important Omega 3 oils, which are good for the heart, prevent inflammation and help keep cells more fluid and healthy.

3. Brazil nuts
High in selenium, one of the most powerful antioxidants.

4. Watercress
Contains antioxidants such as lutein, zeaxanthin and beta-carotene, which are essential for healthy eye function and preventing age-related macular degeneration, which is a disease of the retina that causes loss of central vision.

5. Avocado

Avocados help lower cholesterol and have a cancer-protecting effect. They contain a substance called mannoheptulose that prevents the uptake of glucose into cancer cells. Cancer cells use glucose as their main fuel, so by blocking the uptake of glucose into cancer cells it is essentially starving those cells.

6. Cruciferous vegetables

Include broccoli, cabbage, Brussel sprouts and cauliflower. They have general cancer-protective effects, especially for breast cancer.

7. Garlic

Known for its beneficial effects on blood pressure, cholesterol, circulation, diabetes and cancer.

8. Water

Water helps the body to detoxify by removing waste products, pollutants and toxins.

9. Turmeric

A member of the ginger family, it is a powerful antioxidant and an anti-inflammatory. Helps heart function and prevents hardening of the arteries and is also linked to prevention of cancer.

10. Green tea

Contains powerful antioxidants called polyphenols. Studies have shown that green tea helps to protect DNA from damage and has the ability to ward off cancer.

CHAPTER 5

LIFESTYLE CHANGES

Your diet may be the foundation of your health but you can ensure that its effects are even more powerful now and in the future by making simple changes to your lifestyle.

Some lifestyle recommendations are things you will have already thought of but there may be other things to consider, such as what cookware you use and how you store your food. These can make a significant difference to your health and will only require a small change to what you are doing already.

SLEEP

People in the West are sleeping less; the time we sleep each night has reduced from nine to seven-and-a-half hours since the 1900s. Sleep is important for your health because it gives your body time to recharge its batteries and repair cells and tissue. When you are sleep deprived or aren't getting enough quality sleep you can feel irritable, suffer from poor concentration and, of course, tiredness. The most common problem I see in the clinic is women feeling tired all the time and some can feel tired even if they do sleep well. The tiredness is often a symptom of not enough and/or disturbed sleep and by treating the sleep problem the tiredness goes.

Unfortunately, stress and lack of sleep can become a vicious cycle, because the less sleep you have, the less able you are to cope physically and emotionally with the demands of everyday life and the more stressed you feel (tired but wired). This then makes it harder to get a good night's sleep and you can feel trapped in this never-ending cycle.

Sleep can be more of a problem as you go through the menopause because of symptoms such as night sweats. Some women I see at the clinic are being woken up three to four times a night with night sweats and sometimes they are not able to get back to sleep for over an hour after each episode. For a case study about dealing with night sweats please see page 3.

In this section I am going to cover the effect of sleep on your general health and what you can do to improve the quality and quantity of your sleep, no matter what stage of the menopause you are in.

Sleep is almost seen as a luxury, especially for women, because we feel we can pack more into the day if we sleep less. This might seem logical because you will have more hours awake but when you deprive yourself of sleep you may find that you are not as productive the next day and that lack of sleep will have long-term consequences on your health. The benefits of good sleeping habits are more than just old wives' tales – they're well documented. Good quality sleep has been proven to provide countless benefits to daily life – including a strengthened immune system, increased memory, a trimmer waistline and improved reaction time.

THE BENEFITS OF GOOD SLEEP
Good sleep helps you look and feel better
People who have less than five hours' sleep a night tend to have more physical ailments, such as headaches and stomach upsets and also undergo changes in metabolism similar to those occurring with normal ageing. No wonder many of us look worse for wear after a poor night's sleep! You can spend a fortune on anti-ageing skin creams but you

need to sleep well to have healthy, glowing skin. When you're fast asleep, the body goes into repair mode and regenerates skin, blood and brain cells, as well as muscles.

Good sleep helps you live longer

There is a clear connection between good sleep and disease. For example, according to one study, when deep sleep is interrupted it affects the body's metabolism and reduces its ability to convert sugar into energy, heightening the risk of diabetes.[1] The study found that just three nights of disrupted sleep can have the same effect on the body's ability to control blood sugar levels as putting on more than 2 stone/12.7kg in weight.

Other research shows that those who sleep five hours or less a night are twice as likely to suffer from hypertension (high blood pressure) and heart disease as those who sleep for seven hours or more. Sleeping better may also help you fight off infection. People who don't sleep well often have raised levels of stress hormones and a decrease in immune function.

Inadequate sleep lowers our immune response. One study showed that missing even a few hours a night on a regular basis can decrease the number of 'natural killer cells', which are responsible for fighting off invaders such as bacteria and viruses.[2] This will come as no surprise to those of us who succumb to colds and other illnesses when we are run down – normally after periods of inadequate sleep.

Good sleep helps you lose weight

People who are sleep deprived have an increased appetite. Inadequate sleep lowers levels of leptin, a hormone that suppresses appetite, and increases grehlin, a hormone that increases food intake and is thought to play a role in long-term regulation of body weight. All this suggests that sleep deprivation can make weight loss extremely difficult because it causes your body to work against you!

A large study of nearly 70,000 women conducted over 16 years found that those who slept less than five hours a night gained more weight over time than those who slept for seven hours a night. The researchers also found that levels of exercise did not interfere with the results.[3]

Quality sleep isn't a cure-all and of course you have to combine it with healthy eating and regular exercise, but sleep may have more to do with successful weight loss and weight management than previously thought possible. So before you blame that diet programme for failing, look into your sleep habits and aim for a good night's sleep.

Good sleep makes you smarter

Lack of sleep can have effects similar to those brought on by too much alcohol. Those with sleep deprivation suffer from reduced concentration, memory loss and are more likely to make mistakes and have a slower reaction time. The performance of someone who has been awake for 17 hours straight is about the same as if they had a blood alcohol level of 50mg/100ml of blood (two alcoholic drinks in an hour).

And night owls beware! A study by Harvard Medical School found that people who slept after learning and practising a new task remembered more about it the following day than people who stayed up all night learning the same thing. Better sleep means better concentration and better decision-making.

Good sleep makes you a nicer person

The most potent effects of sleep deprivation are on behaviour. Lack of sleep will make you cranky, aggressive, forgetful and unsociable. Taken to extremes, severe sleep deprivation causes depression, disorientation and paranoia.

DON'T OVERDO IT

Simply put, there is just no substitute for the benefits of sleep. It makes you look and feel healthier, happier, sexier – even thinner! But there's no need to overdo it. Research suggests that oversleeping – and long lie-ins at the weekends – may do more harm than good, as this upsets your biological clock, giving you symptoms like jet lag. So stick to the recommended seven to eight hours; get up at roughly the same time each day – even at weekends – and if you feel that you need to catch up on sleep go to bed earlier rather than sleeping in.

HOW TO SLEEP WELL

Quantity and quality are very important: most adults need between seven-and-a-half and eight-and-a-half hours of uninterrupted sleep. Try to get the best sleep you can by paying attention to your bedtime routine and sleeping environment.

Keep a regular sleep routine

Bedtime routines are helpful for good sleep. Keep routines in your normal schedule. Many women I see tell me they are actually falling asleep around 9 p.m. and then find they are waking too early in the morning. Try to go to bed at the same time and get up at the same time every day. A cup of herbal tea, such as chamomile, an hour before bed can begin the routine. Getting up at the same time is most important.

Exercise

Thirty minutes' exercise during the day can help you sleep better but avoid exercising near bedtime as it can be stimulating. Exercise also delays the production of melatonin, which is known to help with sleep.

Avoid all stimulants in the evening

These include chocolate, caffeinated soft drinks and caffeinated teas and coffee. The effect will be to rev you up when you want your body to calm down ready to switch off for the night. Some women find they can't drink any caffeine after lunchtime as it affects them in the evening and others are so sensitive that just one cup of coffee in the morning has a lasting effect for the day. You need to experiment to see whether caffeine is affecting you. If you are very sensitive then you may find that you can't even drink decaffeinated coffee as there are other stimulants still left in the coffee even though the caffeine has been removed.

Avoid bright light around the house before bed

Using dimmer switches in living rooms and bathrooms before bed can be helpful.

Have a 'to do' list

Write down what you need to do the next day at least an hour before bed. The aim is to stop the dialogue in your head, which can prevent you from getting off to sleep or else wake you up in the middle of the night thinking about something that has to be done the next day.

Keep your bedroom comfortable and restful

Pay attention to the temperature in your room and make sure it's not too warm and not too cold. Cooler is better than warmer. Keep the room restful: a quiet, dark, cool environment sends signals to your brain that it is time to wind down.

Invest in a good bed: if your bed or mattress is uncomfortable or more than 10 years old it may need replacing.

Have a bath

A warm (not hot) bath can help you feel more relaxed. Adding some essential oils such as lavender, chamomile, marjoram and bergamot to your bath can aid that feeling of relaxation. A few drops of these oils can be sprinkled on your pillow and lavender is especially good for this.

Have an orgasm

Sex or masturbation can help to relieve tension and help you go off to sleep faster.

Don't put up with snoring partners

If your partner snores encourage them to sleep in another position or experiment with nasal strips and other snoring remedies. If this doesn't work consider wearing ear plugs or sleeping in a separate room.

Know that the nightcap has a price

Alcohol may help you to get to sleep but it will cause you to wake up throughout the night. While you are sleeping it can make your blood sugar drop, leading to a release of adrenaline and causing you to wake. Alcohol has a diuretic effect on the body so it can also wake you to go to the toilet but also leave you very thirsty. Alcohol also stops the passage of tryptophan into your brain (see below) and it is this amino acid that is converted into serotonin, the 'feel good' brain chemical.

Use relaxation or visualisation techniques

If you find that your mind will not shut off then you need to retrain it to calm down as you go to bed. Sometimes the easiest way to do this, especially if you have an active mind or are a 'worrier', is to think of something else. Take yourself off to a wonderful beach or a beautiful garden and let all your senses become involved. Hear the sounds on that beach, smell the flowers in the garden, feel the sand through your toes, picture the blue sky and really make the place come alive. Each night that you do this, you will find that the time it takes to go to sleep will get shorter and shorter because going to this beautiful place signals to your brain that this is the time for sleep.

Use herbs

Gentle sedative herbs that are the most useful in helping you to sleep include chamomile, valerian and skullcap. Do not use these herbs if you are taking sleeping tablets. It is much better to see your doctor about weaning yourself off sleeping tablets and, at the same time, examine what you are eating and drinking which may be affecting your sleep. Your body goes through different stages of sleep and these stages are important. For the first two-thirds of the night you will have both deep and light sleep and in the last third of the night you will only have light sleep. Throughout the night REM (rapid eye movement) sleep occurs every 90 minutes. Unfortunately, sleeping pills can affect how you go through these stages and can also make you feel drowsy the next day. Of course you should see your doctor before stopping them, but it would be good to address the cause of the sleep problem so that you don't need to take them.

Take magnesium

This mineral is known as 'nature's tranquilliser' and has a calming, relaxing effect on the body in general. It is particularly helpful if your sleep is being disturbed by cramps as it is a muscle relaxant. Take 200mg daily with your evening meal.

Eat tryptophan-containing foods

Your body needs this amino acid in order to make serotonin, the relaxing and calming brain neurotransmitter. Many antidepressants, such as Prozac, are called Selective Serotonin Reuptake Inhibitors (SSRIs) and they work by helping to keep serotonin levels high in the brain.

Tryptophan occurs naturally in certain foods (see list overleaf) so you can use them in your evening meal to help you sleep.

Tryptophan is one of a number of amino acids broken down from the protein you eat. But there are fewer tryptophan molecules in food than the other amino acids and it is easy for the tryptophan molecules not to get into your brain because they are competing with the other amino acids to get through.

If you follow the recommendation of always having protein with carbohydrate (as mentioned on page 34) to keep your blood sugar levels stable, this changes everything. The insulin released when you eat carbohydrates is used by the other amino acids so the tryptophan can get across the blood/brain barrier.

Tryptophan-containing foods include:

- fish
- whole grains
- beans such as soya, chickpeas
- almonds
- peanuts
- eggs
- bananas
- dates
- organic dairy – but add in moderation because of the saturated fat content.

CASE STUDY: DO YOU WAKE AT 3 OR 4 A.M.?

This is a really important question as you go through the menopause and emerge the other side because it can affect women of any age and it is easy to blame it on the menopause. Some women can go back to sleep easily whereas others can be awake for an hour or two once they have woken up, which then has a knock-on effect on their energy and well-being the next day.

A while back a lady came into the clinic in her early sixties, waking with sweats in the middle of the night that were so extreme she had to change her night clothes as they were so damp. She was on HRT, her doctor had even increased the dose and it was still not making any difference to the night sweats. This is really when you have to ask the question 'Are these really menopausal night sweats or are they being caused by something else?' This woman was 10 or so years past the menopause and taking HRT, so logically you would think that all those symptoms would be over by then.

As it turns out, she was not eating well, missing meals and using coffee and chocolate as quick fixes to keep going. She had also been under a huge amount of stress, which had been going on for a while. I recommended that she eat more healthy foods, little and often, and wean herself off the 'quick fixes'. I also put together a good programme of vitamins, minerals and herbs to cushion the impact of the stress on her adrenal glands. The night sweats stopped completely within a couple of months and she came off HRT as it was not helping anyway.

If you find yourself waking with night sweats you want to be clear whether you have woken because you are sweating or you wake and then start to sweat. If you are woken by the sweat then you are having a menopausal night sweat and need to follow the recommendations on page 135 to get rid of them. But if you wake and then start to sweat or get other symptoms such as palpitations or just feel wide awake then this is most likely caused by an adrenaline surge because your blood sugar has dropped during the night, which was the case with the patient above. Follow the recommendations on pages 47–53 to keep your blood sugar in balance during the day and for a couple of weeks while you are changing your diet and getting used to eating little and often, have a small snack of complex carbohydrates, such as an oat cake, or half a slice of wholemeal or rye bread, about an hour before bed. This will stop your blood sugar dropping overnight, and prevent adrenaline from being released into your bloodstream and causing you to wake.

COOKWARE

You might think this an odd topic to include in a book on the menopause but my priority – as well as helping you through the menopause transition easily and comfortably – is also to improve and maintain your long-term health.

When I give talks and seminars, women often ask me what I eat and how I cook my food. My philosophy of using natural solutions for women's health translates not only into food and nutritional supplements but also into how that food is cooked and what it is cooked in.

Using the right kind of pots and pans to cook your food in is really important, because the actual surface of the pan that you are using can end up being absorbed into your food, and subsequently consumed by you. The type of cookware that concerns me most is non-stick. This includes not only pans but also utensils such as food slices that may have a non-stick coating.

Non-stick coatings are applied to metal utensils to prevent food from sticking and to protect cookware surfaces. Perfluorooctanoic acid and its salts (PFOA) are widely used in the manufacture of non-stick coatings. An independent science review panel in the US has recommended that PFOA be considered 'likely to be carcinogenic' based on laboratory studies in rats. The US Environmental Protection Agency (EPA) has also determined that PFOA is 'likely' to cause cancer in rats. While this does not necessarily mean that PFOA causes cancer in humans, I personally do not believe it is worth the risk.

Research indicates that most Europeans and Americans have trace levels of PFOA in their bodies but researchers still aren't sure if this enters via chemicals used in non-stick pans and/or via environmental pollution. Either way, to reduce the risk of the non-stick coating eroding or flaking into your food use only a low or medium heat and avoid using abrasive cleaners, metal scourers or metal utensils when cleaning them. Overheated non-stick pans can also emit poisonous fumes so never leave dry or empty non-stick pans on hot burners.

It also seems that adults with the highest PFOA levels from blood samples were twice as likely to have thyroid problems so these PFOA may have broader health implications.[4] My recommendation, and what I do at home, is to avoid any non-stick pans or utensils completely as it is just not worth having the possibility of that toxic exposure in the house when there are enough toxins coming in from the environment, and it is just as easy to cook with stainless steel or cast iron.

ALUMINIUM

No definite link has been proven, but aluminium has been associated with an increased risk of Alzheimer's disease. I would advise against cooking with aluminium pots and pans and using aluminium foil and cases. Also during cooking, aluminium dissolves most easily from worn or pitted pots and pans so wash and use any you do have with care. Bear in mind too that the longer food is cooked or stored in aluminium, the greater the amount that gets into food. Leafy vegetables and acidic foods, such as tomatoes and citrus products, absorb the most aluminium. People used to cook rhubarb (a very acidic fruit) in an aluminium pan to 'clean up' the pan, which it did very nicely, as the aluminium was neatly absorbed into the rhubarb.

COPPER

Having small amounts of copper coming off your pans and going into your food can be fine for your general health. The problem would be if you were consuming large amounts on a daily basis. Just make sure that if you have copper-coated pans (which haven't been coated with another metal to prevent contact between copper and your food) that you don't use harsh scourers that could wear away the surface and allow the copper to get into your food.

STAINLESS STEEL AND CAST IRON COOKWARE

Stainless steel and cast iron pans are excellent choices for cooking. They are long lasting and put up with a great deal of wear and tear. Cooking acidic food such as tomatoes in an iron pan can be a source of dietary iron and studies show that cooking any food in an iron pot can increase iron intake.

Iron is essential to produce red blood cells. Large amounts can be poisonous, but most women, especially if they suffer from heavy periods, are more likely to lack iron than have too much. Iron cookware provides less than 20 per cent of total daily iron intake – well within safe levels.

CERAMIC, ENAMEL AND GLASS

Ceramic (pottery), enamel or glass cookware is easily cleaned and can be heated to fairly high temperatures. The only health concern about using glassware or enamelware comes from minor components used in making, glazing or decorating them, such as pigments, lead or cadmium. These materials are harmful when absorbed by the body so just make sure you buy a reputable brand as some cheap pans or even dishes have glazes that can contain lead or cadmium in the glazing.

PLASTICS

You should aim to minimise your use of plastic containers and food wrap in general. With plastic wrap (cling film), the concern is that food may absorb some of the plasticiser, the material that helps make it flexible. This is most likely to happen at high temperatures, when microwaving (a cooking method that I don't recommend) or with

MICROWAVING

There are concerns with microwaving food, both about the possibility that radiation could be leaking out while the microwave oven is on, but also that this method of cooking could alter the molecular structure of the food. In a microwave oven the food is agitated over 2,000 times per second and the food effectively heats itself. This process can generate the production of free radicals (see page 75), which are linked to heart disease, cancer and premature ageing.

fatty or oily foods such as cheese and meat. Avoid visibly damaged, stained or unpleasant smelling plastics and containers; never heat food in plastic and if you must buy food wrapped in plastic always remove the plastic when you get home. At home, you can store food in the fridge in a dish with a saucer covering it instead of using wrap or putting it in a plastic container.

SILICONE COOKWARE

Silicone is a synthetic rubber that contains bonded silicon (a natural element that is very abundant in sand and rock) and oxygen. Cookware made from food grade silicone has become popular in recent years because it is colourful, non-stick, stain resistant, hard-wearing, cools quickly and tolerates extremes of temperature (up to 220°C/428°F). There is no known health hazard associated with use of silicone cookware and it is therefore an excellent choice for cooking.

HORMONE-DISRUPTING CHEMICALS IN YOUR ENVIRONMENT

Xenoestrogens ('foreign oestrogens') are oestrogen-like chemicals usually from pesticides or plastics that have been linked to disruptions in hormones for both men and women. These endocrine- (hormone) disrupting chemicals (or EDCs) are chemicals in the environment that mimic our own natural hormones. They are found in everything from plastics to pesticides, and the residues of hormonal medications such as the Pill and HRT that don't break down once they pass into our water supply. Even though the government tells us EDCs are perfectly safe there is a growing body of evidence to suggest that they are not and that they have potentially damaging effects to hormonal health and health in general. In the wild, some of these problems have been dramatic. For example, the Environment Agency has found that a third of the male fish in UK rivers have become feminised and have produced eggs after developing female sex organs.

The increasing levels of xenoestrogens in our environment have coincided with an earlier onset of puberty, with some girls as young as eight starting to develop breasts. Overweight women can have higher levels of xenoestrogens as they are stored in body fat.

I believe it's no coincidence that the huge proliferation of xeno-estrogens in the last 20 years has coincided with a decrease in sperm counts of 50 per cent; an increase in testicular cancer; an increased number of boys born with undescended testes and other problems with their reproductive organs; more girls than boys being born; and an increase in oestrogen-dependent health problems such as breast cancer, endometriosis and fibroids.

DIOXINS

Researchers have found a connection between dioxins (a class of xeno-estrogens from pesticides) and the development of endometriosis. One study found that 79 per cent of female rhesus monkeys spontaneously developed endometriosis after being fed food containing dioxins.[5] Dioxins can be found almost everywhere, not only in the food we eat but also in many products we use on a daily basis, such as the material used for tea bags and sanitary products. Where possible, try to buy organic cotton for products such as sanitary towels and tampons.

In 2006 in the UK two companies had to remove their cod liver oil capsules from the shelves because of the high levels of dioxins (above the legal limit) found in them. In the sea, fish accumulate toxins, which pass through their livers (the organ responsible for detoxification). Extracting the oil from the liver of the fish is likely to provide high quantities of these toxins. My advice is to avoid fish liver oil, such as cod liver oil, altogether and use fish oil taken from the body of the fish. (In my clinic I use Omega 3 Plus from www.naturalhealthpractice.com.)

EXAMPLES OF XENOESTROGENS

Nonylphenols: used in the manufacture of plastics, skin creams, detergents, toiletries, lubricants and spermicides

Bisphenols: leached from polycarbonate plastics especially when heated, for example ready-made meals in plastic trays to be heated in the microwave or babies' feeding bottles

Phthalates: found in make-up, nail polish, hair spray, plastics, carpets

WHAT CAN YOU DO?

- Use plastic wrap (cling film) and containers made of polyethylene, which doesn't contain plasticisers. If the product doesn't make this clear, don't buy it. Avoid polycarbonate (can be marked PC or with the number 7) and also polyvinyl chloride (PVC or with a number 3).
- When you reheat or cook food, particularly in the microwave, don't let plastic wrap touch it. Avoid food that needs to be microwaved in a plastic container. Better still, avoid microwaving food altogether as it changes the structure of the food because of the way it is heated.
- Don't wrap food in plastic wrap; use greaseproof paper instead. Immediately remove plastic wrap from food you buy and transfer it to a glass container.
- Don't store fatty food in plastic wrap. Xenoestrogens are lipophilic (fat loving) and will tend to leach into foods with a high fat content.
- If you buy hard cheese wrapped in plastic, use a knife to shave off the surface layer so you don't actually eat the part that's touched the plastic.

- Use glass bottles. Refill your own non-plastic water bottle instead of using toxic plastic water bottles. While it's good for your health to carry your own water and drink it throughout the day, if it's in a clear polycarbonate plastic bottle, it can be leaching a toxic substance into your water, even if the bottle is sitting on the table at room temperature.
- Buy organic where possible, as this will limit your exposure to pesticide residues. If you are on a limited budget, peel non-organic fruit and vegetables.
- Reduce your intake of saturated fats; meat contains xenoestrogens from the animal.
- Increase your intake of fibre, which helps your body effectively eliminate foreign oestrogens.
- Eat more cruciferous vegetables, such as broccoli, Brussels sprouts, cabbage and cauliflower. They contain a substance called indole-3-carbinol, which will help your body eliminate excess oestrogen.
- Avoid using pesticides in the garden and flea sprays for pets.
- Buy 'natural' cleaning products for your home so you are reducing you and your family's exposure to xenoestrogens. Or better still, make your own – they can be made simply from natural ingredients such as bicarbonate of soda or vinegar. See the following box for more information.

RECIPES FOR NATURAL CLEANING PRODUCTS

Here are some recipes for safe and natural cleaning aids you can make at home.

- **All purpose cleaner:** White or distilled vinegar is a mainstay of old folk recipes for cleaning, and with good reason because it can kill bacteria, mould and germs. Keep a clean spray bottle filled with white or distilled vinegar in your kitchen near your cutting board, and in your bathroom to use it for cleaning. You could also spray the vinegar on your cutting board before going to bed at night, and there's no need to even rinse; let it set overnight. The smell of vinegar dissipates within a few hours.

- **Window cleaner:** One of the most popular recipes for non-toxic window cleaning is white or distilled vinegar and water and you can dry the windows with old newspapers afterwards. You may have found that this formula leaves streaks because commercial products used previously on the glass may have left a wax build-up and vinegar alone won't remove the residue. If this is the case, add a dab of liquid soap to the vinegar and water. Make a great all-purpose window cleaner by combining a quarter of a cup of vinegar, half a teaspoon of liquid soap or detergent and two cups of water in a spray bottle. Shake to blend.

- **Toilet cleaner:** Ditch the bleach. Spray the rim with vinegar and water mix and pour vinegar and two spoons of baking soda in the bowl. Leave for 15 minutes before brushing, then flush.

- **Natural mould remover:** Spray with equal parts vinegar and water mix, leave for five to ten minutes and wipe clean. Fragrant essential oils such as lavender and clove are natural antiseptics and also good at clearing moulds and fungi in the bathroom or on windowsills.

- **Rust remover:** To remove rust scour with cream of tartar.

- **Surface cleaner:** Bicarbonate of soda is a great surface cleaner and shifts stubborn odours. Simply sprinkle a little on to a damp cloth before using.

- **Oven cleaner:** Avoid commercial cleaning products that expose you to unnecessary synthetic chemicals that can add to your body's toxic load. Apply a paste of equal parts salt, baking soda and water to the walls of the oven. Leave for a while (overnight is good) then wipe off.

- **Air fresheners:** Most shop-bought air fresheners do no such thing. They work by using nerve-deadening agents to stop you detecting smells. They are also one of the most concentrated sources of poison in the home and studies have shown that people who use them have more headaches and skin allergies. Make your own real air freshener by adding ten drops of essential oil to a 200g box of baking soda and placing in a dish. You can also clear the air with houseplants, which freshen the air by absorbing the carbon dioxide and releasing oxygen. Plants that reduce toxic materials are: aloe vera, English ivy, fig trees, chrysanthemum, spider plants, Chinese evergreen, bamboo palm and lily.

For natural cleaning products go to www.naturalhealthpractice.com. I have checked the brands listed on this site for harmful ingredients so you do not have to.

TOILETRIES

Your skin is the most absorbent organ of the body so be careful what you rub on it. Take particular care around your breasts because there are oestrogen mimics that could stimulate breast tissue. It is estimated that a woman can end up putting over five hundred different chemicals on her skin each day. Think about the products you regularly put on your skin, from moisturisers and make-up to deodorant and perfume and try to rethink your approach – do you really need or want all these chemicals entering your bloodstream? Can you reduce your 'toxic load', either by reducing the amount of toiletries you use or by buying natural or organic products?

You may be surprised to know that some products that claim to be natural are actually not always as pure as they seem. Some compounds used as ingredients can be derived from a natural substance, but once synthesised in the laboratory are completely artificial. An example is cocomidopropyl betaine which is often cited as a natural substance made from coconuts but is actually synthetic.

There are potentially harmful ingredients in the majority of the personal care products on the market, so as you change to healthier eating and are avoiding chemicals like additives and preservatives in your food, think about the ingredients in the other products you use on a daily basis.

I recommend checking ingredients' lists properly and where possible sticking to natural plant-based products or making your own.

GET TO KNOW THE NASTIES

Products will give you a list of ingredients on their labels. The following substances are the ones you should watch out for.

Formaldehyde: Preservative. Found in nail polish, nail hardeners and other cosmetics. Commonly associated with adverse skin reactions.

Imidazolidinyl urea: Preservative. Commonly associated with adverse skin reactions.

Artificial fragrance: Found in synthetic fragrances, parfum, and used in cosmetics. Be aware that artificial fragrances can often consist of many ingredients and these ingredients do not have to be listed separately on the packaging. Nineteen per cent of children with eczema are fragrance sensitive. Many other studies link rising levels of dermatitis in recent years with an increased use of fragrance chemicals. Phthalates (pronounced THAL-aytes) are allergens found in certain fragrance chemicals and nail varnishes; many are now restricted in use by the EU.

Parabens: Widely used preservatives. Known as methylparaben, propylparaben, butylparaben, ethylparaben. Associated with skin irritation. Some possibility that they may be a xenoestrogen and linked to a risk of breast cancer.

Isopropyl alcohol: Anti-bacterial agent obtained from petroleum (sometimes used in antifreeze). Prolonged contact with isopropyl will result in dry, split skin, headaches, dizziness, depression and nausea.

Methylisothiazolinone: Preservative. Associated with allergic reactions and irritation.

Paraffin: Used in cold creams, hair removers, eyebrow pencils and other cosmetics. Derived from petroleum or coal. Can cause irritation and make the skin more dehydrated.

Propylene glycol: Moisture carrying agent used in cosmetics. Usually derived from petroleum, although it is possible to derive it from vegetable glycerine. Can irritate the skin, lungs and eyes.

DEA (diethanolamine), MEA (monoethanolamine), TEA (methylolamine): Look out for names such as cocamide DEA or MEA or lauramide DEA. These are hormone disrupters and are known to form cancer-causing nitrates in the body. They are almost always found in products that foam.

Mineral oil: This is used in many body lotions (baby oil is 100 per cent mineral oil) and coats the skin like a plastic wrap, disrupting the skin's immunity and not allowing it to breathe or release toxins. Allowing toxins to accumulate results in abnormal cell development, premature skin ageing, acne and other skin disorders.

Polythylene glycol (PEG): This is a preservative, surfactant and skin conditioning agent that actually alters and reduces the skin's moisture levels. PEG increases the appearance of ageing, and allows the skin to be more vulnerable to bacteria.

Sodium lauryl sulphate (SLS) and sodium laureth sulphate (SLES): Strong detergents found in most foaming bathroom products. SLS and SLES are thought to be the most dangerous of all ingredients in toiletries. Research has shown that if SLS combines with certain other chemicals used in the manufacture of toiletries, they can produce carcinogens that stay in the body for up to five days and leave residual levels in the heart, liver, lungs and brain. This potentially could lead to cancers of all these organs. SLS and SLES have been connected to skin irritation, diarrhoea, breathing problems, depression and eye damage.

Triclosan: An anti-bacterial and anti-fungal found in products including liquid soaps, washing-up liquid, toothpastes, deodorants, anti-bacterial chopping boards, shaving gels and some toys. It is thought to cause hormone disruption in the body and, in pregnant women may disrupt the flow of blood to the womb, starving a baby's brain of oxygen and causing brain damage. The EU's Scientific Committee on Consumer Safety is concerned that Triclosan can cause resistance to antibiotics.

NATURAL PRODUCTS

Because you don't have the time to wade through long, complex lists of ingredients on every product to ensure what you buy is natural, organic, safe and effective, I have designed a classification system that enables you to know at a glance how natural a product is.

On the Natural Health Practice website there is a section called 'Natural Beauty Products' that lists products from a number of different companies. I have grouped the products into four classifications of Gold Seal of Approval, Silver Seal of Approval, Bronze Seal of Approval and Nearly Natural Seal of Approval. For more information go to www.naturalhealthpractice.com.

NATURAL HOMEMADE TOILETRIES

Here are some natural, chemical-free recipes you can try at home.

Relaxing bath: Wash away petrochemical perfumes and take a botanical bath. You can have a luxurious relaxing bath that won't dry out your skin by adding natural substances to warm bathwater, such as aromatherapy oils like lavender, rose or ylang-ylang. You can choose different oils to match your mood – for example, lavender has a calming and relaxing effect, while lemon is stimulating and invigorating. Use natural soaps (available from www.naturalhealthpractice.com).

Muslin face soak: Soak a muslin cloth in warm water laced with several drops of essential oil such as rose or lavender. Wring out and press to your face, inhaling the calming properties. The heat oxygenates and the cloth loosens dead skin cells.

Oatmeal skin scrub: Make a paste with a teaspoon of finely ground oatmeal (available from health food shops) and a little water. Use it to gently wash your face, avoiding the eye area.

Avocado mask: Mash and sieve an avocado then mix in a few drops of lemon juice (to stop it discolouring) and a teaspoon of liquid honey. Apply to skin, leaving on as long as possible. It softens, moisturises and nourishes.

Lemon hair rinse: To increase shine when washing fair hair, use a lemon juice solution in your final rinse (one part lemon to eight parts water).

Hand treat: Rub lemon juice over your hands and elbows to soften, clean and bleach them. Rinse fingernails and hands daily in a lemon rinse (but keep away from cuts).

Teeth cleanser: Rubbing sage leaves across the teeth cleanses them and sweetens the breath. Try making your own toothpaste by mixing 2 tablespoons of salt with 3 tablespoons of bicarbonate of soda. Chew cloves to sweeten the breath.

PART TWO

GOING
THROUGH THE
MENOPAUSE

CHAPTER 6

HAVE YOU STARTED TO GO THROUGH THE MENOPAUSE?

When women talk about going through the menopause they are actually describing the perimenopause, which is quite a recent term. It is during this stage that you could experience most of the classic menopausal symptoms but it can start very subtly.

Many women will start to experience hormonal changes from around the age of 40. Some women will notice changes from their mid thirties onwards. These changes can be so subtle that you may wonder if it is all in your mind but rest assured that what you are feeling is completely normal.

When you will enter the perimenopause is difficult to predict and does not seem to depend on when you started having periods, whether you have been on the Pill or how many times you have been pregnant. One definite factor is smoking; being a smoker can push you into the perimenopause one or two years earlier than women who don't smoke.

Having a hysterectomy without having the ovaries removed can give a woman a 50 per cent chance of going through the menopause within five years of having the surgery.[1] If you have been sterilised you may also experience the menopause earlier than women who haven't.[2]

For both hysterectomy and sterilisation it is thought that the change in blood supply to the ovaries after the surgery causes the menopause to happen earlier.

Having a baby when you are 'older' can also tip you into the peri-menopause. One of my patients was in her early forties when she gave birth. She realised that while she was breastfeeding she was starting to get hot flushes. As she reduced the breastfeeding she only had a couple of periods and then went straight into the menopause. The huge hormonal upheaval of the pregnancy just tipped her over into it.

Something like a sudden shock or trauma, such as a car accident or bereavement can also have a dramatic physiological effect. Unfortunately, if you are of a menopausal age this kind of trauma may lead to the sudden onset of menopause.

PREMATURE MENOPAUSE/PREMATURE OVARIAN FAILURE

A premature menopause, medically known as premature ovarian failure (POF), occurs before the age of 40 and occurs in 1 to 4 per cent of women. There may be a definite cause for POF such as radiotherapy but in the majority of cases, up to 70 per cent of women, there will be no medical reason.

A woman could have been having regular periods for a number of years and then suddenly they stop; this can even happen to women in their twenties. This is why, if a woman comes into one of my clinics with amenorrhoea (no periods), I would always suggest that she has investigations. It is very easy to let things slide and not bother about having tests because it is actually more convenient not having periods. But there are health implications such as risk of osteoporosis if this lack of periods is caused by POF.

Don't be fobbed off if your doctor suggests investigations are not necessary. Push for tests to be done as I have seen women who have been misdiagnosed or where investigations have been delayed for years. The menstrual cycle can cease for a number of reasons, including polycystic ovary syndrome, low body weight, stress and pregnancy, but also POF, so it is important to have blood tests to look for high FSH levels and an ultrasound scan to know for sure what is happening.

For most young women it is a very emotional and traumatic situation to be told that they are menopausal and will be experiencing symptoms associated with older women such as hot flushes, night sweats and vaginal dryness. It is so important to get good advice on how to look after yourself and also emotional support if you are given this diagnosis. The UK charity The Daisy Network (I am one of the patrons, see www.daisynetwork.org.uk) supports women with POF and as well as the advice and help that they give, it is also beneficial to know that there are other young women in the same situation as you are.

It is important to get emotional help and support as well as medical advice if you are diagnosed with POF because issues will arise that need to be addressed. There can be a real sense of loss and bereavement. You may also want to discuss fertility choices and these can include egg donation, adoption or to stay positively childless.

I discuss hormone replacement therapy (HRT) in chapter 11 and believe women who experience menopause at the usual age should not use it because it tries to replace hormones that are naturally declining. However, because with premature ovarian failure you are replacing those hormones that your body really *should* be producing the issue is different. The biggest risk without those female hormones circulating is that of osteoporosis so my recommendation would be to replace those hormones in the most natural way possible, for example with bioidentical hormones (see page 182), until you get to the age of around 50. Then you could make the decision to come off those hormones gradually, thus mimicking a 'natural' menopause.

Note that all the health risks talked about with HRT, such as breast cancer, are associated with women taking these hormones later in life, not with women with POF. You have a medical condition; you are not going through a natural stage in your life at the right age, so the same HRT risks do not apply to you.

Not matter what your age I would still suggest that you have these important tests if you have POF (see pages 193 and 273):

- Bone density scan
- Bone turnover test
- Vitamin D test
- Omega 3/6 ratio
- Lipid – cholesterol check

Have these tests done as soon as possible after getting the diagnosis, as the results will then give you a base line from which to make a comparison later on and to keep track of your health.

If you have recently been given a diagnosis of POF then do get in touch with one of my clinics. There may be the possibility of restarting your cycle, especially if your ovaries look healthy on an ultrasound scan (see Useful Resources on page 283).

WHAT ARE THE MENOPAUSE SYMPTOMS?

These can vary from woman to woman and they can be new symptoms, which you haven't experienced before, or some problems like

PMS could become worse. Here are some of the symptoms you might experience:

- sleep disturbances
- anxiety with no discernible cause
- inability to concentrate
- forgetfulness
- PMS
- mood swings
- changes in cycle length (shorter or longer)
- bleeding more or less
- less vaginal lubrication
- lower sex drive
- some hot flushes or night sweats.

The closer you are to your last ever period (the actual point of 'menopause') the stronger the symptoms can be. But if you use the natural solutions in this book you can eliminate them and the sooner you tackle them the better.

WHAT HAPPENS DURING THE PERIMENOPAUSE?

This is an interesting question because everybody assumes that as we get close to the menopause we will have low levels of oestrogen, but in fact during the early stages of the perimenopause there can be parts of your cycle where your oestrogen levels can be quite high.

Let's have a look at the change in your female hormone cycle during the perimenopause.

As you enter the perimenopause you can still be having periods but not ovulating. This is because your egg reserve is lower and your ovaries may not be responding to FSH (follicle stimulating hormone which triggers egg release) as efficiently as before. In an attempt to compensate for the lack of response your body produces more FSH from the pituitary gland, so you have higher levels of this than usual.

When you have a cycle where you do not ovulate, you will not produce progesterone in that cycle. This is usually produced by the corpus luteum, which is formed when an egg is released. Without this, there is no progesterone.

The ovaries may still produce a good level of oestrogen, which means you will have a constant level of oestrogen without the usual balance of the progesterone. If the oestrogen stays quite high you could go 8 to 10 weeks without a bleed, as there is no progesterone to trigger the period.

Oestrogen levels can be affected not only by these hormone changes but also by the amount of foreign oestrogens (xenoestrogens) in your environment (as explained in Part One). High levels of oestrogen at this time have led to the marketing of many products containing 'natural' progesterone in order to offset this imbalance. In order to counteract too much oestrogen ('oestrogen dominance'), promoters of such products state, you need more progesterone.

Symptoms connected to a higher oestrogen to progesterone ratio are anxiety and tension, breast tenderness, headaches, irregular bleeding and water retention.

These same symptoms can also be connected to having low levels of oestrogen, which can occur during some cycles when the follicle does not develop properly. This causes the ovary to release less oestrogen. The LH (luteinising hormone) surge is therefore not triggered and the egg is not released so there is no ovulation.

This illustrates how variable the hormone levels can be during this perimenopausal stage. It is difficult to predict what level they are and they can vary from month to month. The number of days between cycles can increase or decrease, the bleeding can be heavier or lighter, longer or shorter and you can even start to miss some periods. Some periods you will ovulate, others you won't.

If your cycle is very different from how it has always been it is important to get a check-up with your doctor to rule out more serious concerns. This is especially important if the bleeding pattern seems very different. Look out for:

- very heavy bleeding
- bleeding more often than every three weeks
- bleeding that lasts longer than a week
- bleeding between periods
- bleeding after intercourse.

CAN A TEST CONFIRM YOU ARE IN THE PERIMENOPAUSE?

You can have a blood test to see whether you are in the menopause by measuring both FSH and oestradiol (the oestrogen produced by the ovaries). Your doctor can arrange this or you could contact my clinic if you encounter problems (see Useful Resources on page 283).

A high level of FSH could indicate you are in the perimenopause. During the perimenopause, your declining egg reserve means your ovaries need more FSH than usual to stimulate egg development. The body responds to this, resulting in a high level of FSH. It is also important to measure oestradiol when you test for FSH levels because an oestradiol level over 180pmol/l (80pg/ml in the US) will artificially give a lower FSH level. You can get a more accurate measure of your FSH when your oestradiol level is low.

In women before the perimenopause, FSH levels would normally be less than 10iu/l. Any level over 30iu/l can indicate that you are in the perimenopause. However, do not rely heavily on this result because the FSH can vary from cycle to cycle during the perimenopause.

FSH and oestradiol can fluctuate from one cycle to the next and cycles can be irregular in perimenopausal women. It is always best to take the FSH and oestradiol measurement on the second or third day of your period, since at the beginning of the cycle the FSH should be at its lowest, so you will get a truer reading of its real level. A high reading at this time could indicate you are in perimenopause.

If you have had your blood test on day three and the oestrogen (oestradiol) level is high (over 180pmol/l) then you need to repeat the test even earlier in the cycle, for example on day two, to get a true reading of the FSH.[3]

Another way to check what is happening to your cycles and ovulation is to have an ultrasound scan in the first half of the month as this can actually look at the developing eggs (antral follicles) to see whether you are ovulating and show you the size of the ovaries – they get smaller the closer you are to the menopause. It is important to have a scan especially if you have some unexpected bleeding patterns. The scan can also show the thickness of the womb lining: if it reveals that your womb lining has thickened – a condition called endometrial hyperplasia – you will need to get this treated medically because if left untreated the cells could start to mutate and put you at risk of womb (endometrial) cancer.

Scientists are also looking into a test that can predict when the menopause will occur. The ovaries produce a hormone called anti-mullerian hormone (AMH), which helps the eggs mature each month. The fewer eggs left in the ovaries (ovarian reserve) the lower the level of AMH. This hormone is often tested for women going for fertility treatment. But scientists are now working on the theory that the menopause is triggered by AMH falling below a certain level and research has shown that the age of menopause commencement could be predicted from a mathematical model using AMH levels.[4]

At the moment, the mathematical model is not available for general use but we do test FSH, oestradiol and AMH in my clinic. If you can't get the hormones tested locally then do get in touch as they can be organised by post (see Useful Resources on page 283).

Q&A

Can I get pregnant during the perimenopause?

The answer is definitely yes and if you don't want to get pregnant then you must take precautions. The difficulty is that during this perimenopause stage your periods are likely to be irregular. For instance, you could have missed three cycles and then on the fourth cycle you ovulate two weeks before the period would be due. You could then become pregnant on that cycle and not even realise it because you would think that you are just missing another cycle.

Also, to be clear, a blood test that shows high levels of FSH does not mean that you don't need contraception. Your levels are going to fluctuate widely in the perimenopause so although high levels mean you may be menopausal, and your fertility may be lower than before, it does not mean you cannot get pregnant.

You will not need any contraception if you are under the age of 50 and have not had any periods for two years, and you only need one year clear if you are over 50.

What is the best choice of contraception?

I would not recommend the contraceptive Pill because of the possible side effects including, ironically, lower sex drive and decreased vaginal lubrication. Other side effects can include nausea, vomiting, headache, thrombosis, skin pigmentation, depression, bloating and breast tenderness.

From the nutritional viewpoint, the Pill will also deplete your body of valuable nutrients. One of the main ones is folic acid[5] and it is known that there is a link between not having enough folic acid and abnormal changes in the cervix.[6] In one test, when folic acid was given to women on the Pill, abnormal cell changes in the cervix reverted back to normal.[7]

As well as the depletion of folic acid, other nutrients such as the rest of the B vitamins and zinc can become deficient if you are on the Pill. It is known that the B vitamins, B1, B2, B12 as well as folic acid have a protective effect against abnormal cell changes in the cervix.[8]

From the medical viewpoint, the Pill could be used to regulate the erratic cycles during this perimenopause stage but I would recommend natural solutions instead (see page 135). The Pill will mask your menopausal changes, making it difficult to know whether you have reached the menopause so it is normally suggested that a woman should stop taking it when she is 50. The Pill does not delay the menopause; it just prevents you from being able to see what is happening because you will be having a withdrawal bleed from the Pill.

There is no point doing blood tests for FSH and oestradiol while you are on the Pill, as the hormones in the Pill will influence the results.

Medically it is suggested that women who smoke should not take the Pill after the age of 35 because it increases the risk of heart disease and strokes.

The positive benefits from the Pill are the regulation of the cycle and there is a reduced risk of ovarian, womb and bowel cancer, but an increased risk of both cervical[9] and breast cancers.[10] In fact, the Pill can increase the risk of breast cancer by 44 per cent, so at a time in your life when the breast cancer risk can be higher because you are getting older, I would be extremely careful about choosing the Pill as contraception.

Of course, there are other contraception choices, including progestogen-only pills, the ordinary coil (IUD), the coil that releases progestogen (IUS), sterilisation and barrier methods such as condoms. If you are starting a new relationship then do use barrier methods because the risk of sexually transmitted diseases is still a concern.

The coil which releases progestogen directly into the womb is often used during the perimenopausal stage, as it can help when the bleeding is heavy and of course also acts as contraception. It can reduce the blood loss by up to 90 per cent.[11] For some of my clinic patients who have opted for this coil rather than controlling the symptoms naturally, it has worked extremely well and over time they stop having any bleeds. They are not menopausal but the influence of the hormone progestogen has stopped the womb lining building up so it does not have to shed.

On the other hand, there are women where the intermittent bleeding and spotting, which are side effects of this coil in the first few months, does not stop in the long term and they find that they can almost be bleeding all the time. The other most common side effect from this coil is the mood swings. Remember it is the same hormone that is used in the Pill for the second half of the cycle and the one that is linked to mood swings and depression. But when it is being released in a coil, progestogen is not there just for two weeks in the month like in the Pill, it is there every day, and the mood swings and depression can be there constantly.

If you start taking HRT (see page 175) for the perimenopausal symptoms, it will not act as contraception because you can still be ovulating, especially when you first start taking it.

CHAPTER 7

WHAT TO EAT AND
WHAT TO AVOID

Making sure that you are eating well during the perimenopause is not only going to help you with this transition but it will also give you a really good foundation for your long-term health. You may have another 30 to 50 years to live, so you want to take advantage now of sowing the seeds of good health.

Follow the Twelve-Step Hormone Balancing Diet as described in chapter 2. The closer you can follow the 12 steps the better as each of the steps gives you different health benefits.

Pay particular attention to adding phytoestrogens to your diet (Step 1, page 20) as these foods will help cushion the effects of the hormone roller-coaster as you go through the perimenopause. We know that women who eat a diet rich in phytoestrogens have significantly fewer hot flushes, up to half the amount experienced by women who eat very few phytoestrogens[1] so make sure these are included in your diet and go for variety. Don't base everything around soya; include also chick-peas, lentils, flaxseeds (linseeds) and kidney beans (see page 281 for a list of foods that are classed as phytoestrogens).

If you are suffering from increased mood swings, irritability and depression then taking measures to balance your blood sugar is absolutely crucial (Step 12, page 47). This means not only thinking about the quality of the food that you eat but also the timing. You need to completely eliminate added sugar and refined carbohydrates in order to see a marked improvement in your moods.

The other important consideration is to eat little and often. This means not going more than three hours without eating. If you wait longer than this, your blood sugar will drop and the stress hormones adrenaline and cortisol will be released. It is the release of these hormones that gives rise to many of the symptoms relating to anxiety, tension, crying spells, depression and irritability.

Many women can feel a hot flush coming over them as soon as they feel anxious. They may be running late for an appointment or just realise they've forgotten something important and suddenly up comes a hot flush. Hot flushes are connected to your adrenal glands – as your ovaries decline in the production of oestrogen your adrenal glands take over some of this role and produce a form of oestrogen to help protect your bone health. You should therefore aim to reduce the amount of stress hormones your adrenal glands release and this can be done in two ways.

Trying to reduce the stress from outside (see page 78) is not always easy and the only way you may be able to control what is happening is to manage how you react to the stress. The other way to regulate the stress hormones is to watch what and how you eat. Adrenaline and cortisol are released as your blood sugar drops so you can reduce how stressed you are actually feeling by changing what you eat. You may not always be able to control the stress going on outside yourself but you can definitely control what you put in your mouth.

Aim to have breakfast, lunch and dinner and then a small snack in the middle of the morning and one in the middle of the afternoon. By having good quality food, little and often during the day, you can keep your blood sugar levels stable. This not only keeps your weight down but it also boosts your metabolism, gives you more energy and can help avoid Type 2 diabetes by preventing high blood glucose levels, which cause your pancreas to pump out ever-increasing levels of insulin.

CHAPTER 8

HOW SUPPLEMENTS AND HERBS CAN HELP YOU

It is very important to get your supplements and herbs right when going through the menopause because they can make such a difference to how you feel physically and emotionally. You may have to take a few more supplements each day than you did before the menopause but bear in mind that this will only be for a short period of time until you are free of symptoms. After that you should aim to take a maintenance programme of supplements to keep you well as you go through the menopause.

FOOD SUPPLEMENTS

The way to structure a good supplement programme is to take a multi-vitamin and mineral specifically designed for the menopause as the foundation. This will give you 'a bit of everything' including good levels of antioxidants such as vitamins A and E and the minerals zinc and selenium, B vitamins, vitamin D, calcium, magnesium, chromium, manganese and boron (the one I use in the clinic is called Meno Plus, see www.naturalhealthpractice.com). To this you should add in separate supplements of vitamin C and Omega 3 fatty acids.

Vitamin C is an important anti-ageing antioxidant and there will never be enough in a multivitamin and mineral, so you need to take it separately. It is a water-soluble vitamin, which means that it is excreted in the urine every few hours and can't be stored, so it is better to take two doses in one day rather than one large dose. We can't manufacture vitamin C in our bodies so we have to get it from our diet and in supplement form.

Vitamin C is also important for your immune system but its value is even more important as you go through the menopause because it is crucial for the manufacture of collagen. Collagen makes up 90 per cent of your bone matrix so getting enough vitamin C is vital for your bone health.

Omega 3 fatty acids are also added in separately because they are not usually included in a multivitamin and mineral and, if they are, the levels will not be high enough. These are important for their anti-inflammatory action because as your oestrogen levels start to reduce, for some women the main symptom can be painful joints. These fats also help to keep your skin and hair feeling soft, as well as helping with mood swings. They also have a beneficial effect on hot flushes and have been shown to be three times more effective in reducing hot flushes compared to women taking a placebo.[1]

With all this in mind, your Perimenopausal Supplement Programme should involve the following:

- a good high quality multivitamin and mineral designed for the menopause
- 500mg vitamin C twice a day (as ascorbate, not ascorbic acid)
- Omega 3 fatty acids (containing 770mg EPA and 510mg DHA per day).

(The ones I recommend to my patients are: Meno Plus, Vitamin C Plus and Omega 3 Plus, available from Natural Health Practice, see Useful Resources, page 283 for details.)

For tips on choosing a multivitamin and mineral and food supplements, see pages 56–57.

PMS OR MENOPAUSE?

For many women the most difficult part of this stage is the differentiation between PMS symptoms and perimenopausal symptoms. The symptoms may seem identical but it is the timing that is important.

PMS/PERIMENOPAUSE SYMPTOMS

Physical symptoms	Emotional symptoms
Food cravings	Irritability
Water retention	Crying spells
Weight gain	Anxiety and tension
Aches and pains	Forgetfulness
Tiredness	Low self-esteem
Lack of sex drive	Lack of concentration
Changes in sleep pattern	Depression
Bloating	Mood swings
Breast discomfort	Indecisiveness
Palpitations	Fearfulness

Up to 150 symptoms can be related to PMS so it can't be differentiated by symptoms. Whether your symptoms are PMS or perimenopause is dependent on when they occur. Normally for PMS your symptoms would occur after ovulation (approximately the middle of your monthly cycle) and then stop as the period arrives. The difficulty at the perimenopause is that your periods may be irregular or you could be having a gap with no periods for a couple of months, so you can't tell when the middle of the month is.

The best way to deal with this is to keep a diary or chart of your symptoms and note the days on which they occur. Then when your period arrives you can look back at the diary. If your symptoms were mainly only there in the two weeks or so leading up to the period they are premenstrual symptoms. And there will be certain periods of time when you have no symptoms at all and have good energy levels and steady moods. If there is no pattern to when the symptoms come and they seem to be there all the time, then these are perimenopausal symptoms.

There is always the possibility of having a combination of both PMS and perimenopausal symptoms. Were this to happen, what you would see in your diary are certain blocks of time when symptoms seem to be more extreme and magnified. You may be having underlying peri-menopausal symptoms and then for a couple of weeks, before a period comes, suffer from PMS.

You may also have noticed from the box above that there is no mention of hot flushes or night sweats. These are very definitely peri-menopausal symptoms that would occur randomly and are not linked to your cycle.

It is important to know whether you are experiencing PMS, peri-menopausal or even a combination of both symptoms to help tailor the best supplements and herbs for yourself. Be aware that if you are taking HRT (see page 175), it has been found that HRT can cause symptoms that are identical to PMS, caused by the progestogen part of the HRT, which could make your symptoms worse.[2]

The medical approach to PMS is to suppress the cycle either by drugs or surgery. One of the prescription drugs is called danazol, which is a synthetic weak male hormone that prevents ovulation.

Unfortunately it can have side effects such as nausea, headaches, dizziness and, ironically, mood swings, which is one of the PMS symptoms you are usually aiming to eliminate. As danazol is a male hormone it can also result in other symptoms such as increased facial hair, acne, weight gain and increased sex drive.

Another drug approach is to use GnRH (gonadotropin-releasing hormone) analogues that work directly on the pituitary gland and stop the release of both FSH and LH, effectively putting you into a drug-induced menopause, by stopping ovulation and the menstrual cycle. But because these GnRH analogues are triggering the menopause they cause menopausal symptoms such as hot flushes and night sweats, as well as other side effects such as mood swings, vaginal dryness, headaches and insomnia.

To counteract these 'menopausal symptoms' the standard approach is called 'add-back therapy' whereby HRT in some form (usually tibolone) is given at the same time as the GnRH analogues. You take a second drug to counteract the side effects of the first drug.[3] None of these prescriptions address the underlying cause of the problem; they just suppress the symptoms.

One other drug approach is to give an anti-depressant because many of the PMS symptoms are mood related. However, the anti-depressant is often prescribed to be taken all the time when the symptoms are only occurring for a week or two each month.

The surgical approach is to remove the ovaries, based on the same logic as the drugs – that if you are not having a cycle you can't have PMS. This is the most radical treatment possible – it is irreversible and often the womb is removed as well as the ovaries. One medical article called it 'the only effective cure for PMS',[4] which I would have to totally disagree with. After the surgery you are given HRT in the form of oestrogen to protect your bones.

But the point that is really important here is that there are no differences in hormone levels between women with PMS and women without.[5] The problem is not the hormones themselves but the woman's sensitivity to her own hormones.

In one study, two groups of women, one group with PMS and one group of non-PMS sufferers, were given a drug to 'switch' off their menstrual cycle. The women with PMS found their symptoms were eliminated on the drug. They then gave both groups of women oestrogen, progesterone or a placebo on separate occasions. For the PMS sufferers, it did not matter whether they were given oestrogen or progesterone, the symptoms returned within a couple of weeks. For the women without PMS they noticed no change when given either hormone or placebo.[6] We need to address why these women are reacting to their female hormones rather than just shutting them off completely with either long-term drugs or drastic surgery.

My approach for addressing PMS/perimenopause symptoms is to get you into good health so no matter what hormonal fluctuations your body goes through it can deal with them easily and comfortably. This means that you need to follow the Twelve-Step Hormone Balancing Diet (see page 18) and at the same time add in some key nutrients and herbs on top of the Perimenopausal Supplement Programme from page 128.

SUPPLEMENTS FOR PMS SYMPTOMS

If you think that most of your symptoms are actually premenstrual ones then you need to add in the following extra nutrients.

Vitamin B6

Take 50mg in total as pyridoxal-5-phosphate, so if you have 25mg in your multivitamin and mineral you only need to add in an extra 25mg.

Magnesium

You need 200mg daily, but there should be enough in your multivitamin and mineral.

Zinc
Take 25mg daily but check how much is in your multi before you add in extra.

HERBS

Herbs can be particularly helpful when you are aiming to get your hormones back into balance. It is better to take a combination of herbs as these can give you a quicker effect than taking herbs singly. The best combination I have found for PMS is agnus castus, black cohosh, skull-cap and milk thistle. You take the combination over a period of three months while also following the Twelve-Step Hormone Balancing Diet. (The dosages below are when taken in a combination.)

HERBS FOR PMS
*Agnus castus (***Vitex agnus castus***)*
This is the herb of choice for premenstrual symptoms. It has been found to have a balancing effect on the female hormones.[7] Its effects have even been compared to an anti-depressant for the severe form of PMS termed premenstrual dysphoric disorder and there was no statistically significant difference between how well the drug worked versus the herb.[8] When there is a natural solution that works equally as well as the drug it seems logical to use the natural remedy.
Dose: 200–400mg per day.

*Black cohosh (***Cimicifuga racemosa***)*
This herb is particularly helpful for the anxiety and tension symptoms of PMS, and also the headaches and migraines that occur premenstrually.
Dose: 140–280mg per day.

Skullcap (**Scutellaria lateriflora**)

While the agnus castus is working on hormone balance, the skullcap together with the black cohosh has a calming effect on your body.
Dose: 80–160mg per day.

Milk thistle (**Silymarin marianum**)

Milk thistle improves liver function. It is your liver that has to detoxify your female hormones so you want it to be working efficiently.
Dose: 60–120mg per day.

Follow this programme for three months along with eating well and you should be able to stop the herbs after that time because your symptoms will have gone.

(The organic combination of these herbs that I use in the clinic is called Agnus Castus Plus available from www.naturalhealthpractice.com.)

NOTE

In 2010, new herbal regulations were put in force so that certain herbs such as agnus castus, black cohosh, skullcap and milk thistle need to be licensed and are now only available from limited sources (for example, www.naturalhealthpractice.com, or see Useful Resources page 283 for contact information).

The other alternative is to use herbs that are now listed as foods rather than medicinal herbs. I recommend a combination of vitamins, minerals and herbs including the B vitamins, magnesium, chromium, Siberian ginseng, chamomile and dandelion (see NHP's PMSupport Plus at www.naturalhealthpractice.com).

SUPPLEMENTS AND HERBS FOR PERIMENOPAUSAL SYMPTOMS

If you are suffering from hot flushes, night sweats and other peri-menopausal symptoms follow the Perimenopausal Supplement Programme on page 128 and then add a combination of herbs, black cohosh, agnus castus, dong quai, sage and milk thistle in the quantities given below.

Many years ago in the clinic, I would just use one herb at a time and it was interesting that two women with identical symptoms given the same herb could have completely different responses; one woman would find the herb very effective and the other would report that it had no effect on her symptoms at all. I would then need to try another herb with the second woman. Accordingly, over the years I have found that giving a combination of herbs helps the majority of women in the shortest possible time.

I am going to go into quite a bit of detail with the herbs because I know from the questions that women ask me in the clinic and at talks that you need to know what you are taking and why. The herb with the most research behind it is black cohosh.

Black cohosh (Cimicifuga racemosa)

This is the herb of choice for the menopausal symptoms of hot flushes and night sweats and there have been a number of good clinical trials that show its effectiveness. The majority of studies indicate that 'extract of black cohosh improves menopause-related symptoms'.[9] If you are getting mood swings and anxiety black cohosh can also be helpful for these symptoms of the perimenopause.[10]

Black cohosh does not increase oestrogen levels and has no effect on the cells in the vagina or womb.[11] This is important because this is where the risks are with HRT; it increases oestrogen levels and stimulates tissue in various places in the body including the womb and breast and therefore can increase the risk of cancer. Black cohosh offers relief

135

from menopause symptoms without oestrogen-like effects.[12] More-over, when scientists put black cohosh together with oestrogen-sensitive breast cancer cells they found that the herb actually slowed down the rate at which the cells multiplied.[13]

So how does black cohosh work on the menopausal symptoms if it is not having an oestrogenic effect? It is actually working as a SERM (selective oestrogen receptor modulator). These are substances that can stimulate oestrogen receptors in some parts of the body and not others. So they can block stimulation in places like the womb and breast where it would be unsafe to have cells over-stimulated but they can stimulate oestrogen receptors in other places where you would want stimulation such as the bones and brain. These SERMS are able to target cells appropriately. In contrast, HRT works by simply replacing hormones.

SERMs are the new drug alternatives to HRT (see page 217) but nature already supplies us with SERMs in the form of black cohosh and foods like phytoestrogens (see page 24). A SERM such as black cohosh can help relieve menopausal symptoms without the risk of stim-ulating cells in a dangerous way.

As well as the benefits on menopausal symptoms further research has shown that black cohosh could have other benefits for women. Research in the *International Journal of Cancer* has shown that black cohosh may halve the risk of breast cancer. The researchers found that the use of black cohosh was associated with a 61 per cent reduction in the risk of breast cancer.[14]

Black cohosh's SERM effect shows that it is acting as an oestrogen promoter in organs where oestrogen is needed, such as the bones, while acting as an 'anti-oestrogen' in organs where unnecessary oestro-gen can be dangerous (for example, the breast and womb). This would explain the beneficial effects of black cohosh on breast cancer because the herb can actually block the oestrogen receptors in the breast.

As one study put it, 'such data suggest a non-oestrogenic or oestrogen-antagonist effect of *Cimicifuga racemosa* (black cohosh) on human breast cancer cells leads to the conclusion that *Cimicifuga race-mosa* treatment may be a safe, natural remedy for menopausal symptoms in breast cancer'.[15]

However, there have been some reports of adverse effects on the liver in the press. A couple of years ago there were concerns about black cohosh and liver disease. This problem is extremely rare and there have only been four complaints compared to the estimated nine million treatment days (as it is termed) purchased each year.

When the European Medicines Agency (EMEA) reviewed all the evidence worldwide, it concluded that it was not clear whether black cohosh caused the problem. The National Institutes of Health in the US believes there's no case to answer and their website states that black cohosh has few side effects and that 'liver damage has been reported in a few individuals using black cohosh, but millions of people have taken the herb without apparent adverse health effects. Studies have not provided scientific evidence to show that the herb causes liver damage.'

So, I still recommend black cohosh as the herb of choice for peri-menopause symptoms but make sure that you buy from reputable companies so that you know you are getting the best quality herb and preferably buy organic. Choose herbs that are not standardised (read the label); this is how they have been traditionally used for centuries.
Dose: 150–270mg per day.

Agnus castus (Vitex agnus castus)
This herb is classed as an adaptogen as it has a balancing effect on your hormones. It works on the pituitary gland, which is the gland that sends the message down to the ovaries to release hormones. Agnus castus can help increase levels of certain hormones if they are too low and decrease them if too high. This is particularly helpful in the peri-menopause years because your hormones can be fluctuating widely and this herb helps to create a kind of stability. It is also the best herb to take if you are getting mood swings, anxiety and tension.
Dose: Up to 300–550mg per day.

Dong quai (Angelica sinensis)

Dong quai is a herb from traditional Chinese medicine and is helpful for both hot flushes and night sweats. It has a long history of traditional use. Research has shown that it not only starts to help reduce the hot flushes and night sweats in one month but is also helpful for fatigue and disturbed sleep.[16]

Dose: 150–250mg per day.

Sage (Salvia officinalis)

This herb, which is also easily used as a tea, is helpful in controlling both hot flushes and night sweats.[17]

Dose: 150–250mg per day.

NOTE

As with the PMS herbs, new 2010 regulations mean that certain herb combinations such as black cohosh, agnus castus, dong quai, sage and milk thistle need to be licensed and are now only available from limited sources. The combination I use (opposite), in my opinion, is the best for combating the symptoms at this stage.

If you are having problems getting these herbs then my supplier of choice for all the different supplement brands I use in my clinics is the Natural Health Practice (go to www.natural healthpractice.com or see Useful Resources page 283 for contact information).

The other alternative is to use herbs that are now listed as foods rather than medicinal herbs. The next best combination I recommend includes fermented organic soya, red clover, hops, sage, dandelion, alfalfa and lignans (see NHP's MenoSupport Plus at www.naturalhealthpractice.com).

Milk thistle (Silymarin marianum)

In any situation where you are aiming to balance the female hormones it is very important to add in herbs like milk thistle, which can improve liver function. It is your liver that is doing the hard work of detoxifying your hormones so you want to make the job as easy as possible.
Dose: Up to 130mg per day.

(The organic combination of these herbs that I use in the clinic is called Black Cohosh Plus. If you have difficulty getting this locally then go to www.naturalhealthpractice.com.)

St John's wort (Hypericum perforatum)

This herb is best known for its help with mild to moderate depression[18] and although it has not been shown to help with perimenopausal hot flushes and night sweats it can improve quality of life and reduce sleep problems.[19]
Dose: 300mg twice a day.

HOW LONG DO I KEEP TAKING THE SUPPLEMENTS AND HERBS?

The supplement programme, including the multivitamin and mineral, vitamin C and Omega 3 fish oils, should be taken for the long term as it works on your general health now and into the future.

With the herbs you should start to see a reduction in your symptoms over the first month and after three months they should completely disappear. The herbs are only needed if and as long as you have the perimenopausal symptoms – once they have gone you can stop taking them. If you are not seeing any difference at all after the first month (even a slight reduction in severity or frequency of your symptoms) then the herbs are not working and you either need to try a different brand of a higher quality, or else get in touch with my clinic for help (see Useful Resources page 283).

HERBS AND HRT

If you decide to take HRT (see page 175) then you should not take herbs at the same time unless you are under the supervision of a qualified practitioner (see below). The aim of the herbs is to control the menopausal symptoms, the same aim as HRT. If you are on HRT and still getting hot flushes and/or night sweats then you should go back and talk to your doctor to ask for a higher dose or different brand, or make the decision to come off it completely.

It is not advisable to add in herbs on top of the HRT to try and address the symptoms. The only exception to this is if you are taking three months to come off HRT (see page 189). You can then use the herbs while you are gradually weaning yourself off HRT.

CHAPTER 9

KEEP MOVING

In the first part of the book we looked at why exercise is very important as you approach and go through the menopause, so you will already be aware of its many benefits in helping to prevent disease and keep you in good health. Refer back to chapter 3, and follow the advice given there on when and how to exercise.

As you go through the stage of perimenopause, exercise is vital in helping you experience a comfortable journey and ensuring a healthy life beyond the menopause. I will cover some important issues here including the effect of exercise on symptoms, brain health, weight loss and osteoporosis.

EXERCISE AND MENOPAUSAL SYMPTOMS

Both the Royal College of Obstetricians and Gynaecologists in the UK and the North American Menopause Society have recommended that women should use exercise to help treat the menopausal symptoms of hot flushes and night sweats.[1] I also recommend natural solutions for these symptoms (see page 135), but it seems that for many women exercise can help with both the physical and psychological symptoms associated with the menopause. If you consider this along with all the other benefits of exercise, you will realise just why it is so important to get and stay physically active.[2]

EXERCISE, MEMORY AND BRAIN FUNCTION

We know that physical exercise strengthens muscles and also that doing mental exercises helps to keep you mentally sharp. But it is interesting to know that physical exercise can also help you mentally.

There has been a great deal of research in the last 10 years to show that your physical activity can help brain function, or cognition as it is more usually termed. One study of a group of women over the age of 65 tracked their level of physical activity over eight years. The researchers found that those women who were the most active had a 30 per cent lower risk of cognitive decline. What was interesting was that it was not the intensity of the exercise that made the difference, but the amount. So with walking, the distance the women walked was more important than how fast they walked. This brings me back to the idea I mentioned in chapter 3 of low level, but frequent exercise, such as housework, and how it can reduce the risk of breast cancer.[3]

Your physical activity during the menopause can have such an impact on your brain function that the effects can be seen up to 21 years later – so exercising when you are between 44 and 58 will benefit you when you are between 65 and 79 years of age. If you just exercise at least twice a week for about 30 minutes, it can reduce your risk of dementia and Alzheimer's later in life. This piece of research showed that the beneficial effect of the exercise was so strong that it was independent of whether the women smoked, drank alcohol or had a family history risk of Alzheimer's or dementia. The women who exercised had a staggering 52 per cent lower risk of having dementia compared to the sedentary group.[4] It is thought that exercise increases blood flow and oxygen to the brain, resulting in improved mental agility.

The interesting aspect of all of this research is that your level of physical activity in your mid-thirties can have an enormous impact on your brain function and memory later in life. If you exercised in your mid-thirties it can help you slow your memory loss when you are between 43 and 53 years of age. But if you stop exercising in your mid-thirties then you lose that benefit. The good news is that if you only start exercising in your mid-thirties then you still get the benefit. The message is that it is never too late to start exercising and becoming physically active, and that whatever you do will give you benefit.[5]

EXERCISE AND WEIGHT LOSS

The tendency to gain weight can be a problem throughout the menopause. The two factors working against you are the drop in oestrogen and the change in your metabolism. As you go through the menopause and your oestrogen levels decline, your body will put on extra weight (fat), especially around the middle because fat is a manufacturing plant for oestrogen and will help to compensate for the loss from the ovaries.

Your metabolism can also decline and this is mostly due to a loss of muscle. After the age of 40, women can lose about 8oz (225g) of muscle a year and between the ages of 40 and 50 about 5lb (2.25kg) of muscle in total can be lost. You may wonder why this matters. Because muscle is metabolically active, the more muscle you have the more fat you burn, even sitting still.

The best way to exercise is to have a combination of physical activity that helps to protect your heart and bones, but at the same time helps you to maintain your weight and body shape. Choose exercises such as brisk walking, dancing, jogging or tennis for your heart and bones, and then also include some weight training (resistance) exercises. The weight training exercises could include lifting free weights such as dumbbells or using the weight machines at the gym. They can also include press ups (on your knees is fine if you can't do a full press up), lunges and squats, which all help to build muscles. Other ways to strengthen your body and muscles include using resistance bands (like large rubber bands), and also gardening and household chores that require lifting and digging. Aim to do these strengthening activities two to three times a week.

Research has shown that women who did weight training over a two-year period were less likely to gain weight around the middle.[6]

If you feel nervous about weight training and it's not something you've tried before, start slowly. If you are a member of a gym ask one of the trainers to show you how to use either the weight machines or the free weights. Technique is important because it prevents any strain on your body and allows you to target certain muscles to strengthen. You may have a local council-run gym you can use as and when you want to without a joining fee; again someone will show you how to use the equipment. Some private gyms offer free day passes so you can see whether you like the gym and would want to join and you may even be able to pay less if you use it at off-peak times.

Weight training exercises can also be done easily at home and free weights are inexpensive to buy. I have covered how to do these exercises in my book *Fat Around the Middle,* or you could buy a DVD (presented by a fitness expert rather than a celebrity).

With weights you should aim to do three sets, each set consisting of lifting the weight 12 times, with one minute's break between each set. You can judge if you are lifting the correct weight for you, because you only want to be able to lift the weight about 10 times when you get to the third set. As you get stronger, if you find you can lift the weight 12 times easily on the last set then that is the time to increase the weight.

You also want to keep yourself flexible as well as strong so it is worth considering a flexibility-boosting form of exercise such as yoga. You may be surprised to hear that yoga can also help keep your weight down. Research has shown that women who practise yoga for at least 30 minutes a week gained less weight than those who didn't.[7] The practice of yoga or Pilates will help you to master deep 'belly breathing' techniques, which can help with stress management. By learning how to breathe deeply, rather than taking the usual shallow breaths, you will increase your feelings of calm and general wellbeing.

You may also find that regular exercise like walking can change your feelings about food and even curb your appetite. Research has shown that when overweight people exercise regularly they produced more of a protein called neutrophic factor, which is thought to help reduce hunger. The overweight people in the study not only had a reduced appetite but also weighed less, had a lower blood pressure and a smaller waist circumference after just 12 weeks.[8]

For more advice on weight loss and management see chapter 10.

EXERCISE AND OSTEOPOROSIS

Osteoporosis prevention is one of the most important reasons to make sure that you keep active on a daily basis as you go through the menopause. In order to keep up your bone density you need to place demands on your skeleton, as it is definitely 'use it or lose it' when it comes to your bones. Vibrating plates have recently been promoted as an effective piece of exercise equipment for preventing and eve reversing osteoporosis (see page 71).

However, any exercise that has an impact and forces you to work against gravity is good for prevention of osteoporosis because it helps to build bone density. So walking is good and other aerobic exercises such as jogging, dancing, step climbing and cross training are also beneficial. Weight training (weight resistance) is also helpful for bone health as it increases muscle mass and because your muscles are attached to the end of your bone, the stronger the muscles become, your bones also strengthen to match the muscle strength. Although swimming is good for your heart it does not have the same bone-building effect as impact/weight-bearing exercise because the water holds up your body weight.

Exercises like yoga, t'ai chi and Pilates help to keep you flexible and to strengthen core muscles in the abdomen. They can also strengthen your bones because, again, they work on the muscles that are attached to the bones. They also help to improve balance and co-ordination. Many exercises are performed on one leg and much of the osteoporosis research is focused on preventing falls.[9] Preventing falls is really important as you move into your fifties, sixties and beyond.

EXERCISE AND YOUR SEX LIFE

As well as all the other health benefits, exercise can help you have a good sex life well into your eighties. At a time when you might be worrying about a reduced sex life as you go through the menopause it is good to remember that exercise keeps you healthy and gives you energy. Research has shown that those people who are healthy are twice as likely to be interested in sex as those whose health is not very good. The interesting part is that for those who are unfit, their sex life can often end some 20 years earlier than for those who are fit.[10]

Another aspect of exercise is that it can make you feel good about your body and that can give you the confidence and self-esteem to feel happy taking your clothes off and being intimate with your partner.

CHAPTER 10

HOW TO CONTROL YOUR WEIGHT

For many women, trying to control their weight is a bugbear all their lives but weight gain can become more of a problem when going through the menopause. I'd therefore like to give you some guidance on how to lose weight in a healthy way, at a time when you might be tempted to shed the pounds by depriving yourself of the valuable nutrients that you especially need at this time.

I also want to cover being underweight in this chapter too, because there are a number of women I see in the clinic who can't gain weight and want to as they are too thin. I will also explain why being underweight is not good during the menopause years.

When I talk about being over or underweight I am really talking about being 'over-' or 'under-fat'. There is a big difference between weight and fat.

I believe that measuring weight or even body mass index (BMI) (a ratio of height to weight) is pointless. It is possible to have an athlete and a couch potato with the same BMI and yet completely different levels of muscle and fat. Muscle weighs more than fat, so a muscular person with very little body fat can weigh quite a lot but will not really be 'fat' even though their BMI could register that they are obese.

NOTE

If you have gained weight unexpectedly it could just be due to the menopause but you should see your doctor to rule out a thyroid problem (see page 161) or a side effect of a medication such as anti-depressants.

OVERWEIGHT

During the menopause you may become aware that you have lost your waist and that extra pounds may be settling around your middle rather than elsewhere on your body. For some women this change in shape from a 'pear' to an 'apple' is the first sign that they are going through the menopause.

Your ovaries produce less oestrogen as you go through the menopause, so your body tries to compensate by making you fatter. Fat around the middle of your body manufactures oestrogen, which can offset the lower levels of oestrogen produced by the ovaries.

Putting on a little extra weight during the menopause stages is fine but it can become a health problem if you have too much fat around the middle.

HOW MUCH IS TOO MUCH?

Your waist to hip ratio should measure less than 0.8. You calculate this by measuring your waist and hips and then dividing your waist measurement by your hip measurement. If the ratio is higher than 0.8 this is not healthy (whatever stage of the menopause you are in) as it increases your risk of cancer (especially breast cancer because of the excess oestrogen being produced), heart disease, high blood pressure, Type 2 diabetes, stroke and Alzheimer's. See my book *Fat Around the Middle* (Kyle Cathie) for more information on this subject.

You must take action to reduce a ratio that is higher than 0.8 because of the long-term health risks. As you get older, your metabolism slows down so it unfortunately requires a different strategy to combat this weight gain, especially if it is targeted in the one area, namely the middle in this case.

LOW-FAT IS NOT THE SOLUTION

The standard thinking is that fat makes you fat and you should therefore reduce your fat intake and buy skimmed milk and low-fat or no-fat foods. But I feel that this message could actually have contributed to the obesity epidemic not only in the UK but also elsewhere, and has caused the health crisis we have in the UK with the prevalence of cancer, heart disease and Type 2 diabetes.

Obesity causes at least 30,000 deaths a year in the UK and the UK Department of Health estimates that one in three adults will be dangerously overweight within 15 years.

It is estimated that the obesity epidemic will double the number of cancer deaths within 40 years because we know that excess body fat is a cause of cancers of the bowel, breast, womb (endometrium), oesophagus, kidney and pancreas.[1]

Type 2 diabetes has risen from 2.6 cases per patient years in 1996 to 4.31 in 2005[2] and the World Health Organisation says that this accelerating rise in Type 2 diabetes could result in the first reduction in life expectancy in 200 years.[3] Diabetes has been described by Professor Sir G. Albert, past president of the International Diabetes Federation, as 'the biggest health catastrophe the world has seen'. And then we have heart disease, which is the most common cause of death in the UK, affecting one in five men, and one in seven women, one of the worst rates in Europe.

I have emphasised all these statistics because with many people buying low-fat products you would think we would be doing better, but the situation is actually getting worse. My research suggests that all these degenerative diseases, as they are termed, are being caused by the same thing; they just manifest differently depending on your own family history. And the key to keeping yourself healthy and preventing these illnesses is also the key to weight loss.

What does the research say about low-fat diets and weight loss?

The opposite of what you would think. A large review looked at all the randomised controlled trials from 2000 to 2007 comparing the effects of low-fat or low-carbohydrate diets on weight loss. People on the low-carbohydrate diets had significantly more weight loss at 6 and 12 months than the low-fat diets. The people on the low-carbohydrate diets also had significantly higher levels of good (HDL) cholesterol and lower triglycerides (blood fats).[4]

LOW-CARB NOT LOW-FAT

The key to weight loss is not a low-fat diet but a low-carbohydrate diet. Not a 'no-carbohydrate' diet, which is unhealthy as your body needs energy from carbohydrates, but a diet in which *quality* carbs are consumed in moderation. It is the quality of the carbohydrates that makes the difference.

This brings us back to the difference between refined and unrefined carbohydrates (including sugar) and the effects these have on your body.

What happens as you eat?

Shortly after eating, your blood sugar is high and insulin is released to move the sugar (glucose) out of your blood and into your cells to be used as energy. Excess blood sugar can be stored as energy in your liver and muscles, ready to be turned back into blood sugar if you need a quick burst of energy.

But this energy storage is very small, so once it is filled up, the excess blood sugar is stored as *fat* in fat cells. As a woman you have about 35 billion fat cells (known as adipocytes) compared to a man's

26 billion, which is a lot of storage space. In addition, fat cells can expand to over a hundred times their original size in order to store more fat if needed.

Insulin is your fat-storing hormone. Anything that causes more insulin to be produced causes more fat to be stored. The foods that increase insulin are the refined carbohydrates (including white grain products such as bread and rice, and foods containing sugar such as fruit yogurts and breakfast cereals, as well as foods containing both white flour *and* sugar such as cakes and biscuits).

It doesn't matter how many low-fat foods you eat – *if your diet comprises a large amount of refined carbohydrates you are never going to lose weight.*

WHY QUICK-FIX DIETS DON'T WORK

Insulin not only tells your body to store your food as fat, it also prevents the body from burning off fat. And the important word here is fat, not weight. For healthy weight loss, you can only lose about 1 to 2lb (0.5 to 1kg) of fat a week. So when a women's magazine has a headline saying 'lose a stone in a month', bear in mind that weight lost that quickly is not fat loss but just water and muscle loss.

As soon as you go back to normal eating after the diet, your body then registers that it has to replenish those fat stores in case another 'famine' happens soon. This means that the weight you lost goes back on as fat and you can end up with more body fat after a diet than before. The next diet has to be even stricter as you have more fat to lose. So it goes on. This is known as yo-yo dieting and it plays havoc with your metabolism.

The biggest key to losing weight is to *stop dieting*. You should aim for a way of eating that is a way of life, where you can eat like that 80 per cent of the time (the other 20 per cent is for holidays and birthdays etc.). You'll find you lose fat healthily and easily, and at the same time you'll be reducing your risk of Type 2 diabetes, heart disease and cancer.

The two most important points to follow are:

- eliminate refined foods
- eat little and often – every three hours.

You want a blood sugar level that comes up gradually because the food is unrefined, which means your body does not have to produce an excessive amount of insulin, and before your blood sugar drops after three hours you have eaten again.

If you commit to eating this way, you will notice four big differences:

1. **You will have more energy:** By stopping the roller-coaster ride of energy highs and lows, you will have a more sustained level of energy for the whole day.

2. **Your cravings for sweet foods and carbohydrates will go:** On the roller-coaster, when your blood sugar drops (known as hypoglycaemia) your body will send you off for a quick fix like a bar of chocolate because it needs to raise your blood sugar quickly. When you are eating unrefined carbohydrates, and eating little and often, your blood sugar does not crash down, so the craving for the quick fix disappears.

3. **You will lose weight (especially around the middle):** As your body does not have to produce high amounts of insulin it does not have to store your food as fat. It stops putting that fat around the middle where it is close to your liver in case it needs to get at it quickly in an emergency.

4. **Your mood swings will disappear:** You will feel much calmer as your body is not releasing adrenaline because your blood sugar is not dropping.

THE NINE WEIGHT LOSS MISTAKES A WOMAN CAN MAKE

She:

- skips breakfast (in an attempt to eat less)
- eats too many refined carbohydrates
- eats too little protein
- thinks all fat is bad
- undereats in the first half of the day
- overeats in the second half of the day
- doesn't lift weights adequately (if at all) – see page 68
- eats too infrequently (meals are way too far apart)
- has her biggest meal at night, often a 'binge' or 'out of control' meal, then wakes up not hungry, skips breakfast and starts the cycle all over again.

SUPPLEMENTS TO HELP YOU LOSE WEIGHT

If you want to lose weight there is no substitute for a healthy way of eating, but there are certain nutrients that can make the whole process easier while you are getting used to your new approach to food.

The aim is to take a programme of supplements for three months and then go on to a maintenance programme. But your first priority must be to shift the excess weight (fat) especially if it is sitting around your middle, no matter what age you are.

The point of taking supplements is to encourage your body to burn off excess fat and to help it respond efficiently to insulin so it does not have to produce too much. At the same time, certain supplements can help reduce the stress hormones, especially if you have been riding the blood sugar roller-coaster.

Chromium

One of the most important nutrients for helping to control insulin levels is chromium. Research has shown that giving chromium supplements to diabetics helps them control the amount of glucose (sugar) in the blood.[5]

Other research has shown that taking chromium supplements helps to not only reduce blood sugar levels in people with Type 2 diabetes but also reduces a substance called glycosylated haemoglobin (HbA1c), which is a measure of how well the diabetes is being controlled (the lower the level in the blood the better).[6]

In summary, chromium can help insulin to do its job properly. Remember, insulin's job is to remove the glucose (sugar) from your blood and move it into your cells. If you can keep your insulin levels low, your body will store less glucose as fat, so losing weight is easier. Chromium also helps cells be more sensitive to insulin so that your pancreas does not have to produce so much of it in order to move glucose from your blood into your cells.

When a grain is refined the chromium content is stripped away. When that refined grain (for example, white flour) is subsequently eaten, the glucose it contains will hit the bloodstream really fast, making it even more important to ensure you have good levels of chromium, to help control the excess glucose and to ensure your blood sugar levels are in balance as far as possible.

Dose: 200µg per day for at least three months. This can be included in a good multivitamin and mineral or taken separately.

The B vitamins

The B vitamins are important nutrients for weight loss as they are needed for glucose metabolism and also play an important role in balancing blood sugar.

Three of the B vitamins (B2, B3 and B6) are important for healthy thyroid function. Vitamin B5 plays a part in turning glucose into energy, instead of fat, and is the most important B vitamin to take if you are under constant stress.

Dose: It is better to take a good B complex (or multivitamin), containing all the B vitamins, rather than taking separate B vitamins. Taking them separately is inconvenient and also likely to be more expensive. You should aim for approximately 25mg of each of the B vitamins per day.

Magnesium

Magnesium has a general calming effect on the body but it also plays a significant part in weight loss because it helps to keep blood sugar in balance. This mineral is also important because it is needed to keep your cells sensitive to insulin. This prevents your pancreas from being overworked by having to produce too much insulin.

One study found that if you have low levels of magnesium you have a 94 per cent chance of developing Type 2 diabetes, which makes this mineral very important not only for helping you to lose weight but also for your future health.[7]

Additionally, being under stress can deplete your magnesium so it can be important to replenish your levels with supplements.

Dose: 300mg per day.

Zinc

This mineral is crucial when it comes to weight loss because hundreds of the enzymes that your body uses depend on it. Zinc is involved in the production of many hormones, including thyroid hormones and insulin, so is crucial for balancing your blood sugar and maintaining your metabolism. Not having enough zinc can actually change your appetite and make you eat more. Taking extra zinc can actually help in the production of a particular hormone called leptin, which is produced by fat cells. Leptin levels are important as this hormone tells us when we have had enough to eat and are full. Researchers have shown that they can increase leptin production just by giving people zinc supplements.[8]

Dose: 25mg per day, either on its own or preferably contained in a good multivitamin and mineral.

Vitamin C

I have included vitamin C as a supplement to help with weight loss even though everybody associates it with the immune system. Vitamin C is needed for glucose metabolism and research has shown that people with diabetes have up to 30 per cent lower levels of vitamin C.[9] It is also thought that a good intake of vitamin C might help regulate blood sugar and help prevent diabetes.[10]

Vitamin C can also give you a bit of an advantage when it comes to keeping fit. If you have adequate levels of vitamin C when you exercise you can burn 30 per cent more fat than people with low levels of vitamin C.[11] Anything that is going to make exercise more effective is obviously especially helpful.

Dose: 500mg as ascorbate (not the acidic ascorbic acid) twice a day. As humans we can't manufacture vitamin C in our bodies so have to get it all from outside and because it is water soluble we can't store it. For this reason, splitting the dose of 500mg is better than taking 1,000mg once a day.

Omega 3 fats

These fats are important for your general health but are especially important for weight loss. Research on animals has shown that Omega 3 fish oils reduce body weight and help burn off fat (compared with Omega 6).[12] Omega 3 fats can improve your metabolism as they play a part in a process called thermogenesis which raises body temperature and helps the body to burn off fat.

Dose: 1,000mg per day with 770mg EPA and 510mg DHA (the one I use in the clinic is called Omega 3 Plus and you only need to take two capsules to get this amount. See www.naturalhealthpractice.com.)

MY 10 GOLDEN RULES FOR HEALTHY WEIGHT LOSS

Rule 1: Never skip breakfast

The old saying that 'breakfast is the most important meal of the day' is certainly on the money when it comes to dieting. Sleep causes your metabolism (fat-burning capability) to slow right down and nothing gets it going faster than breakfast. But always remember that just as important as having breakfast itself, it's also vital to choose healthy breakfast options such as wholegrain cereals like porridge, organic 'live' natural dairy products like yogurt, organic eggs and fruit. Sugar-laden cereals will cause your blood sugar to rise sharply and drop quite quickly – you need something that will sustain you and keep you feeling fuller longer. Porridge is particularly good for this.

Rule 2: Get plenty of sleep

New links between amount of sleep and weight loss are being uncovered all the time. One case in point was a series of studies published in the *Journal of the American Medical Association*, which showed that lack of sleep can make weight loss far more difficult than it needs to be. Make sure your weight loss doesn't encounter any hidden barriers to success by getting plenty of sleep. Aim for seven to eight hours a night.

Rule 3: Eat regularly

Eating little and often will help curb hunger pangs and keep your blood sugar levels and fat-burning metabolism steady, so make sure you have a selection of healthy snacks on hand, such as nuts and raisins, seeds and pieces of fruit. Aim to eat three small to medium-sized meals a day (meals should not be too large because you will also be having snacks), plus two or three healthy snacks. Don't go for longer than three hours without eating.

Rule 4: *Don't try to lose weight too quickly*

Gaining significant weight usually takes years so losing a significant amount of weight can also take time. Our bodies are built to resist sudden and significant change through a process called homeostasis – effectively the body's way of maintaining the status quo. If you try to lose weight too quickly your body automatically slows down its metabolism – the rate at which you burn energy to survive and function – and this is an example of homeostasis at work.

Early rapid weight loss is usually a result of losing body fluid and muscle tissue, which is neither healthy nor helpful in your battle to lose weight. Rapid and significant weight loss from dieting alone is usually indicative of a very calorie restrictive diet, which can be counterproductive because it is often unsustainable and when weight is gained again it goes on as fat. This is because your body perceives the restricted calorie diet as a famine and assumes that it might happen again. To protect itself, it wants extra fat storage just in case. So you actually get fatter after a diet and then the next diet has to be even more restrictive, and this carries on. You should aim for a weight loss of no more than 1 to 2 pounds (0.5 to 1kg) a week; slow weight loss will result in fat loss rather than muscle and water loss.

Rule 5: *Make fruit and vegetables your best friends*

They are full of important metabolism (fat burning) and health boosting vitamins and minerals. Make the most of them (see page 31).

Rule 6: *Keep moving*

Exercise keeps your metabolism up which is why weight training to build or maintain your muscle mass as well as aerobic activity like walking, jogging, cycling and swimming are so important when you want to lose weight. Diet alone is not the best route to weight loss and maintaining an ideal weight range; to lose weight safely and keep it off permanently, always combine healthy eating and exercise. Around 30

minutes of moderate intensity exercise a day is a minimum require-
ment so if you don't want to join a gym, find ways to include more
activity into your life, for example walking more instead of driving or
taking the stairs instead of the lift. You could put on a favourite CD at
home and dance round the kitchen or get a small rebounder (mini-
trampoline). You can even use free weights like dumbbells when
watching the news or your favourite programme on the TV so that
you are making the most use of your time.

Rule 7: *Don't deny yourself the foods you enjoy*

Most diets fail because they call for you to eat foods you may not actually like. If you don't like what you're eating, then clearly you're not
going to stick with your diet for more than a week or two. The key to
successful weight loss is to reduce the amount you eat and introduce
healthier options of the foods you like gradually into your diet over
time. Don't deny yourself the foods you enjoy; if you cut out all the
foods you enjoy your diet is bound to fail. Moderation is the name of
the game when it comes to healthy eating and long-term weight loss.
Think of eating well 80 per cent of the time; the odd blip is not the end
of the world.

Rule 8: *Watch what you drink as well as eat*

As well as helping to keep you healthy, drinking sufficient amounts of
water keeps you feeling full and stops you from feeling hungry, and
when you drink plenty of water you usually drink fewer soft drinks,
coffees and alcohol, all of which can add significant amounts of calories, not to mention additives and preservatives, to your daily intake.

Also be extra careful with those highly calorific flavoured coffees
where you can add cream and even marshmallows; they are literally a
dessert in a cup. And don't go too mad on fruit juices; one glass of
orange juice can contain the juice of eight oranges. Unfortunately,
most of the fibre is thrown away so you are left with a high amount of

fruit sugar hitting your bloodstream fairly quickly with no fibre to slow it down. If you are having a fruit juice, dilute it half and half with water and drink it with food, which will slow down the effect of the fruit sugar. A smoothie would be a better choice because all the fruit (fibre and all) is put into the blender and just whizzed up, so you do not lose anything from the whole fruit.

Rule 9: Avoid extremes of any kind

Balance is not only the key to a happy, healthy life; it is also the key to a healthy diet and weight loss. Be wary of any diets that are very restricted either in the types of food that you can eat or the amount. Diets that are extreme in one way or another are likely to be unhealthy at best and dangerous to your health at worst. If you're ever considering a diet that promises very rapid and significant results, remember that your body is designed to maintain the status quo and the only way to successfully lose weight and keep it off is to make sure you get enough nutrients from a wide variety of foods and to follow a thought-through, realistic weight-loss programme.

Rule 10: Streamline your cooking

Eating well isn't just about the food you choose – how you cook it matters too. Here are some essential bits of equipment that will help you make your cooking tastier and healthier.

- **A set of good stainless steel pans:** They will keep you from using unhealthy non-stick ones. (See page 100 for more information on why you should avoid non-stick pans.)
- **An oil mister or spray:** This delivers a fine mist of oil that is great for lightly coating your pans. It will give your food a crispy texture without leaving it swimming in oil and is great for sautéeing.

- **A steamer:** Up to 70 per cent of vitamins B and C can be destroyed by boiling or overcooking vegetables in large amounts of water. Steaming helps preserve these vitamins and also the colour and flavour of the vegetables.

Bear in mind that if you have a lot of weight to lose, you've got a better chance of success if you get help. Even if your weight isn't directly affecting your health now but you want to get ahead in the battle of the bulge, a nutritionist can help keep you motivated and on track (see my contact details on page 283 if you would like personal help). There may be an emotional component to your eating habits and this may need to be resolved if it is getting in the way of your weight loss.

Finally, don't give up or panic when you have a bad day (because the chances are you will), just start again the next day. One bad day will not ruin your healthy eating plan. Aim to follow my Twelve-Step Hormone Balancing Diet as the basis of your healthy eating plan, and try to eat this way 80 per cent of the time. Don't worry about the 20 per cent blips, everybody has them!

YOUR THYROID GLAND

The thyroid gland is situated in your neck and helps control your metabolism, which in turn controls your weight, so it plays an important role in weight management. Your thyroid produces a number of hormones, the most important being thyroxine (also called T4). Thyroxine, an inactive hormone, becomes activated when converted to triidothyronine (called T3). Your thyroid gland is like a thermostat that regulates your body temperature and tells your body to burn calories and use energy. It is the T3 hormone that makes the metabolism work faster and burn fat.

If you have been gaining weight, it is always important to rule out a medical reason for this. Have a look at the symptoms below and if you can say 'yes' to four or more of them your thyroid gland could be underactive, so you should see your doctor to have your thyroid function tested by a blood test. You will notice that many of the symptoms below can also be symptoms of the menopause so it is really important to know whether they are linked to your thyroid or not.

- Has your weight gone up gradually over months for no apparent reason?
- Do you often feel cold?
- Are you constipated?
- Are you depressed, forgetful or confused?
- Are you losing hair or is it drier than it used to be?
- Are you having menstrual problems – irregular or heavy periods?
- Are you experiencing a lack of energy?
- Are you getting headaches?
- Is your skin drier than before?
- Have you noticed that the outer third of your eyebrow is missing or has got thinner?

TESTING FOR AN UNDERACTIVE THYROID (HYPOTHYROIDISM)

An underactive thyroid is more common in women than men, affecting around one in fifty women, and tends to be most common in women aged over 40. An underactive thyroid is much more common than an overactive one (see page 172).

An underactive thyroid may be caused by one of two things: either your pituitary gland is not producing enough thyroid stimulating hormone (TSH) or your thyroid is not working properly.

A way to test whether you have low thyroid function at home, without a blood test, is to measure your temperature. If your temperature is too low, it may indicate that you have a sluggish metabolism caused by an underactive thyroid.

This test measures your basal body temperature, your body temperature at rest, so you need to be able to take your temperature in bed every morning upon waking. If you are still having periods, then take your temperature on the second, third and fourth day of your period (your body temperature naturally rises as you go later on in the cycle). If your periods have stopped, then take your temperature on any three consecutive days. Take the average of the three results you have and if that average is lower than 97.6°F (36.4°C), it is worth seeing your doctor for a blood test for thyroid function. You could have a low body temperature indicating a sluggish metabolism but not show any thyroid problems from the blood test so medically you would not be offered any treatment. In this case, make sure that you put all the recommendations below (see page 165) into place to try to improve your metabolism.

You may already be taking thyroxine tablets for poor thyroid function but still find that you are not losing weight and your energy has not improved. If this is the case, it is important that you have another blood test to check that you are on the correct dose of thyroid hormone. If you are, then it is really important that you follow the recommendations I give below in order to try and improve your thyroid function as it may then respond more effectively to the medication.

If you find yourself in the situation where you are doing all the right things and the dose of thyroxine is correct but your symptoms still do not seem to be improving then I would suggest that you ask for your T3 level to be checked. This is not routinely done in the UK although it is quite commonly tested in the US. Most of your T3 is converted from T4 so while you may be receiving an adequate dose of T4 it may be the conversion to T3 that is causing problems. If a blood test reveals that the level of T3 is low, then clearly your body is not effectively making the conversion.

Remember, T3 is your active thyroid hormone; its job is to speed up your metabolism and help burn fat, so if your T3 level is low, you won't be getting any of the benefits of the thyroxine on your metabolism, namely extra energy and weight loss. With thyroid hormone testing it is important to know your levels of 'free' T4 and 'free' T3 as these are the unbound and biologically active forms of the hormones. You do not want to measure your total level of T4 as this is bound and the body cannot use it, which is why the free form is so important.

The other way to help with the conversion of T4 to T3 is to consider what a nutritional approach can achieve and to use the dietary recommendations I offer below to improve your thyroid function generally. It's worth paying particular attention to certain nutrients, which can be added in supplement form, that help the conversion of T4 to T3. Selenium, zinc and magnesium are important for this conversion and also a resin called gum guggul from the mukul myrrh tree. (It is best to take all these nutrients combined in one supplement called T Convert. If you have difficulty getting hold of it then do get in touch – see Useful Resources page 283.)

DIETARY RECOMMENDATIONS TO IMPROVE YOUR THYROID FUNCTION

As with so many conditions concerning hormonal imbalance, the first line of treatment is dietary. In general, the better the quality of your diet, the healthier your thyroid gland will be, as will every other gland, organ and cell in your body. If you have not started taking thyroxine and your test results are borderline, following these dietary and supplement recommendations may mean you will not have to take it. If you are already on it following these recommendations may mean you can stay on the lowest possible dose of thyroxine. More specific dietary recommendations are outlined below.

I will start with foods that are unhelpful if you have poor thyroid function. You don't need to cut them out of your diet completely, but foods to eat *less* of are: cabbage, kale, broccoli, kohlrabi, mustard, lima beans, sweet potato, peanuts and soya products. These foods are goitrogens, which means they can block the uptake of iodine (see below) and make thyroid problems worse. These foods only seem to be a problem when they are eaten raw and excessively, so make sure they are cooked well and eaten in moderation.

Since it takes more energy to break down protein than carbohydrate and fat your metabolic rate increases in relation to protein intake. A healthy thyroid diet should therefore be based around eating good sources of protein such as fish, legumes (pulses), eggs, nuts and seeds. An adequate intake of protein will also deter the hair loss that often accompanies an underactive thyroid condition.

A diet that is heavy in alcohol, caffeine and sugar will over-stimulate the thyroid, and this overwork can lead to the thyroid eventually being unable to fulfil its function. Cutting back on sugary foods and drinks, limiting or eliminating alcohol and caffeine and eating a healthier balanced diet will give your thyroid the break it needs to rejuvenate and start working properly or, if you take thyroxine, to enable you to use the thyroxine efficiently and stay on the lowest dose.

SUPPLEMENTS TO HELP YOUR THYROID

In general, a multivitamin and mineral is essential in the thyroid diet (choose one that is appropriate for your age; if you are over 40, then Meno Plus is a good one, see Useful Resources page 283) but the following specific nutrients also help optimise healthy thyroid function.

Iodine

This mineral is a necessary component of T3 and T4. Iodine combines with the amino acid tyrosine and gets converted into the two thyroid hormones. It is well documented that a diet low in iodine is associated with hypothyroidism (underactive thyroid). For this reason, ensuring you get sufficient amounts of iodine from fish, seaweed, shellfish and sea salt is critical for the optimal function of the thyroid. In Japan, the daily intake of iodine from seaweeds is estimated to average 3mg and thyroid disorders are extremely rare in that country. Herbalists have traditionally used the seaweed bladderwrack (kelp), which is rich in iodine, to help with an underactive thyroid. However, I advise you to proceed with caution and consult a qualified practitioner rather than suggesting a generic dose of kelp here – if you take too much iodine you can actually make an underactive thyroid condition worse.

Selenium

Increasing your intake of selenium has also been shown to boost thyroid function as selenium, along with zinc (see below), is essential for the prevention of diminishing T3 hormone levels. T3, remember, is the active thyroid hormone that burns fat. If your T3 levels are low, your metabolism inevitably slows down. You can boost your intake of selenium by eating foods such as wholemeal bread, Brazil nuts, tuna, onions, tomatoes and cooked broccoli. Include some of these foods on a regular basis in your diet.

Dose: 100µg per day in supplement form. Check whether your multi-vitamin and mineral contains this amount and if not you will need to supplement the extra.

Zinc

This mineral is important for the healthy production of your thyroid hormones and also plays a part in appetite control. (See page 153 for supplements to help you lose weight.)

Dose: Aim to get around 25–50mg per day, so add in some extra zinc if your multivitamin and mineral contains less than this.

Manganese
Manganese is important for healthy thyroid function as it is used by enzymes that help to produce the thyroid hormones.
Dose: 5mg per day.

Tyrosine
Tyrosine is an amino acid that is needed in the production of your thyroid hormones. Good 'thyroid' supplements contain mainly tyrosine and the nutrients mentioned above together so that you do not have to take them all separately. Do get in touch if you have difficulty getting them locally (see Useful Resources page 283).
Dose: 200mg per day.

NOTE
If you are taking an iron supplement always take it separately from other food supplements. This is especially important if you are taking thyroid medication as the iron could decrease the absorption of the thyroxine.

EXERCISE
Physical activity is especially important if you suffer from an under-active thyroid because it can help speed up your metabolism and boost weight loss. Brisk walking, so that you are slightly out of breath, for 30 minutes per day, gradually building up to 45 minutes, is a good goal to have in mind. If you already take regular exercise, increase it by an extra 10 minutes to make your body work a bit harder and get the maximum benefit. See page 158 for more tips on exercise.

REDUCE STRESS
Stress is thought to be a contributing factor to the development of hypothyroidism. This is because the high levels of the hormone cortisol

that are released when you are stressed reduce your levels of the thyroid hormone T3. Added to this, high levels of cortisol will urge your body to break down muscle to provide glucose for your brain, and the less muscle you have the slower your metabolism will be. Stress management techniques such as breathing, meditation and yoga are all recommended. Another great way to reduce stress is to take regular exercise. Taking regular time out is also crucial, so make a point of enjoying some 'you time'. Try to balance your life for the sake of your health.

MASTER OF YOUR METABOLISM

Remember, the thyroid hormone is the master metabolism hormone. And even if your thyroid is functioning healthily, eating a healthy diet and exercising regularly can help keep it that way and functioning optimally.

If your thyroid is out of balance, your metabolism is out of balance too and this will make any attempt at weight loss tough. You may be prescribed medication by your doctor, and this can work alongside your new eating habits to help resolve your difficulties. However, in my experience, even while on medication, weight loss is slower than normal, so it is *very* important to stick closely to a healthy eating plan *and* take regular exercise.

CASE STUDY: SARAH'S STORY

Sarah went to her doctor for a routine check-up because she had not been feeling too well. She was constantly tired, to the point of finding it hard to get out of bed in the morning and falling asleep on the sofa at night. She had noticed that her hair was becoming thinner and drier and her skin looked dry and pale. She just put this down to the menopause, but when her blood results came back they showed that she had borderline low thyroid function (hypothyroid). Her doctor recommended that she take a drug called thyroxine. Sarah was reluctant to start this because she had always tried to live a natural life and only used medication as a last resort.

As the result was borderline her doctor said it was okay to postpone the medication if Sarah wanted to try the nutritional approach first.

Sarah then came to my clinic and I asked her to complete a nutritional questionnaire showing what she ate on a daily basis and checked to see if she had any mineral deficiencies. I explained how the thyroid gland works and that the usual thyroid test measures the levels of the two hormones, TSH and T4 (thyroxine). What is not measured, however, is the hormone known as T3 that thyroxine converts into within the cell, which is much more biologically active. For a cell to convert thyroxine into the active T3, selenium needs to be present.

I asked Sarah to eat more iodine-rich foods like fish and to include some seaweed (wakame, dulse and nori). Her mineral analysis confirmed she was deficient in selenium so I also advised Sarah to eat Brazil nuts, oats, brown rice and seafood for their selenium content.

I started Sarah on a programme of vitamins, minerals and herbs to support and nourish her thyroid gland and help with the production of the T4 and T3. She was given a multivitamin and mineral, Omega 3 fish oils and vitamin C for her general health. To this I added extra selenium and a specific formula containing Siberian ginseng (for stress) and tyrosine to help improve the functioning of the thyroid gland.

She came back after six weeks for a follow-up consultation and reported a marked improvement in her energy. She was waking refreshed in the morning and actually getting up on the first alarm. She also felt more energetic in the evening and this enabled her to do more exercise, which in itself gave her more energy. Her hair was also looking thicker and had more life in it.

A blood test after three months showed that her thyroid hormones were back within the normal range but I advised Sarah that she needed to continue looking after her health and to stay on the complete supplement for another three months. After that she could remain on the maintenance programme of a multivitamin and fish oil and vitamin C supplements.

Sarah put in the effort to make changes in her diet and lifestyle but, of course, there are situations where drugs are needed. The problem with thyroxine is that once people start to take it, it becomes incredibly hard to come off it in the longer term as the thyroid gland becomes used to it and ultimately the thyroid could end up working even less efficiently.

UNDERWEIGHT

Many overweight women I see say they would give anything to be underweight. But being underweight is actually just as much a health risk as being overweight.

If you have always been a low weight and it has never stopped your cycle or interfered with you getting pregnant then this is just the way you are made and it is not unhealthy. You may find that you put on a few extra pounds (especially round the middle) as you go through the menopause, which will actually be useful as that extra fat will produce oestrogen, and this can help to protect against osteoporosis.

If you are eating well and are losing weight then you should see your doctor for a check-up to make sure that there is not a medical problem such as an overactive thyroid that is speeding up your metabolism. An overactive thyroid can increase your risk of osteoporosis.

If you lose 10 to 15 per cent of your body weight quickly, especially during the perimenopause, it can stop your cycle and push you into the menopause sooner than you should be.

The other risk of being underweight throughout the menopause is to your bone health. Being underweight or slim framed is a known risk factor for osteoporosis (brittle bones that fracture easily) so this is a good reason *not* to crash diet around the menopause.

If your doctor has checked you and everything is fine but you have difficulty gaining weight then I would always suggest looking at your digestive system.

POSSIBLE REASONS FOR BEING UNDERWEIGHT

Coeliac disease

The first thing to do would be to have a test for coeliac disease. This is an autoimmune condition affecting one in a hundred people in the UK, although it is estimated that many people have coeliac disease and remain undiagnosed. Symptoms can include weight loss, diarrhoea, constipation, bloating and flatulence, mouth ulcers, joint pain and hair loss. It is often mistaken for IBS (irritable bowel syndrome) because of the similarity of the symptoms but it is important that coeliac disease is tested for in order to rule it out.

In coeliac disease, the person's immune system reacts to the gluten in grains (rye, wheat, barley and oats) and damages the lining of the small intestine. This damage to the intestines stops the absorption of valuable vitamins and minerals including vitamins A, D, E, K, folic acid and other B vitamins, zinc and selenium. It will also affect the absorption of calcium if a person is deficient in vitamin D.

If you are suffering from some of the symptoms listed and think coeliac disease may be the cause the easiest way to test for it is to have a blood test. The test will be looking for certain antibodies produced in someone who has coeliac disease when gluten is eaten. If you have problems getting this test done, then contact me (see page 283 for details), as this test can be organised by post. Do not change your diet before doing a test for coeliac as you need to keep eating gluten every day (at least in one meal) for six weeks before doing the test, otherwise it could reveal a false negative result.

Your doctor may refer you to a gastroenterologist who can do a biopsy to check for coeliac disease.

Other digestive problems

You may not be absorbing what you eat properly because you have a different kind of digestive problem, for example a parasitic infection, and a simple stool test can be done to rule this out. The stool test will also look at how well you are absorbing in general and will check for any yeasts or negative bacteria (bacteria that is not beneficial for your health – the opposite of beneficial bacteria). This test also lets you know if you have good levels of beneficial bacteria (which are good for your health) such as lactobacillus acidophilus and bifidobacterium. If you would like to do this test, do get in touch as it can be done by post (see page 283).

Overactive thyroid (hyperthyroidism)

As with an underactive thyroid, hyperthyroidism is more common in women than men. As you might imagine, having an overactive thyroid is the opposite problem to an underactive one and in this case your body is producing too much of the thyroid hormones. This increased thyroid activity will make your body feel like it is in overdrive and it will speed up many of the body's processes.

Symptoms can include:

- weight loss
- loose and frequent bowel motions
- palpitations
- sweating
- increased appetite
- bulging eyes
- anxiety.

It would be a very good idea at any time to see your doctor if you are experiencing a number of these symptoms but it is even more important around the menopause as having an overactive thyroid increases your risk of osteoporosis, heart disease and stroke.

The problem is that because your metabolism works faster when the thyroid is overactive, everything is speeded up, including bone turnover (when your bone builds up and breaks down to replace the bone with healthy new cells), so you can be losing bone faster than you are building it up.

From a medical point of view, the aim is to reduce the thyroid's hormone production either by using medication (an anti-thyroid drug) or by destroying or removing some of the thyroid gland (either by surgery or by taking radioactive iodine (RAI) in pill form or in water). The RAI is used as a one-off treatment and because only the thyroid gland picks up iodine it only affects the thyroid; no other tissue is affected. The RAI causes the cells in the thyroid to reduce or stop functioning so less hormone is produced.

YOUR DIET

What you eat should keep your thyroid functioning as well as possible, along with any medical treatment you might be having.

To help reduce the thyroid hormone nutritionally you should include more raw cruciferous vegetables like cabbage, cauliflower and broccoli in your diet (when raw these can block the uptake of iodine and this blocking is beneficial when the thyroid is overactive as its function is driven by iodine), and reduce foods that are naturally high in iodine such as sea salt, seaweed like kelp and also dairy foods. Note that dairy food itself does not naturally contain iodine but in the milking industry the cows' teats and udders are washed in iodine-containing sanitising agents from which iodine gets into the milk supply. These iodine-containing sanitisers were replaced with other non-iodine containing ones in Australia several years ago and research shows that iodine deficiency is now becoming a problem among people with a normal thyroid function.[13]

SUPPLEMENTS

Take a good multivitamin and mineral in order to keep yourself as healthy as possible. It should contain good levels of magnesium, calcium and vitamin D to help protect against bone loss, which is a risk with an overactive thyroid.

Some nutrients can be particularly helpful for an overactive thyroid problem, including the following.

Vitamin E
This vitamin is a powerful antioxidant and without good levels of this nutrient your body can produce too much thyroid hormone.
Dose: 400–600ius per day.

Vitamin C
Not having enough of this antioxidant vitamin can cause your thyroid gland to produce too much thyroid hormone. As it is water soluble and excreted every few hours through the urine, it is important to have good levels on a daily basis when you have an overactive thyroid.
Dose: 500mg twice daily in ascorbate form (not ascorbic acid).

Co-enzyme Q10
This is an important antioxidant, which is reduced if your thyroid hormone levels increase. It is important to have good levels of this nutrient if your thyroid is overactive as it can help minimise some of the symptoms.
Dose: Aim for 60mg per day.

L-carnitine
Like co-enzyme Q10, this amino acid can reduce some of the symptoms of an overactive thyroid.
Dose: 500mg per day.

Omega 3 fatty acids
Inflammation can cause your thyroid to produce too much hormone and Omega 3 fatty acids, especially EPA, can be helpful in reducing this.
Dose: 1,000mg of fish oil with 770mg EPA and 510mg DHA per day. (The one I use is called Omega 3 Plus and you only need to take two capsules to get this amount. See www.naturalhealthpractice.com.)

CHAPTER 11

HRT AND BIOIDENTICAL HORMONES

My views on HRT (hormone replacement therapy) are quite clear: I believe that the menopause is a natural phase in every woman's life and it should not be medicalised by replacing hormones that should not be there at that stage. The advice in this book is designed to provide you with a foundation of good health before, during and after the menopause using natural, nutritional and dietary aids.

However, HRT is a subject that may come up during any stage of the menopause. You may be at the stage where you need to make a decision about whether to take HRT or not so in this chapter I aim to provide you with all the facts.

It is interesting to note that, since 2003 in the US, HRT has been renamed hormone therapy (HT) omitting the word 'replacement', suggesting that the drugs are risk free, which they definitely are not. It has been acknowledged that HRT does not replace hormones that *should* be there at that time in a woman's life. There is a reason *why* the hormones are on the decline and it is not as straightforward as replacing like for like.

When you are taking any medication the benefits should always outweigh the risks and I believe this is not the case with HRT. If unpleasant symptoms can be controlled with natural remedies – including dietary and lifestyle changes – why take the risk of using HRT, which can incur unpleasant side effects and increase the possibility of a serious illness such as breast cancer?

The only exception to this is when a woman goes through an 'early menopause' (otherwise known as premature ovarian failure) before the age of 40 (see page 115). This is definitely a medical problem and not a natural stage in a woman's life. In this situation, by taking HRT she is really replacing those hormones that *should* be there. All the research detailing the risks of taking HRT that is listed below does not apply to a woman who has gone through a premature menopause. The best approach in this situation is to have regular bone density scans to monitor your bone health (see chapter 12 for more advice) and to take HRT in its most natural form as bioidentical hormones where possible (see page 182 for more information on bioidentical hormones).

RISKS OF TAKING HRT

The main purpose of taking HRT is to control the two major symptoms of the menopause: hot flushes and night sweats. Many women start taking it as soon as the symptoms appear; others might wait and only take it when the symptoms affect their quality of life. It used to be that women could start taking HRT at the menopause and stay on it for ever if they chose but it is now recommended that they only stay on it for the short term (see page 180).

HRT has been around since the 1930s in various forms and over the years has been touted as a miraculous anti-ageing drug designed to transform women's lives during and after the menopause. However, research began to indicate that it was not a miracle drug and that HRT increased the risk of breast, womb and ovarian cancer, heart disease, strokes and blood clots (thrombosis), and gall bladder problems.

Although the risks of taking HRT had been known for some time, it was the US Women's Health Initiative (WHI) Study in 2002 that really changed everything. This study, which involved over 27,000 women, was abandoned after five years instead of continuing for eight because women taking HRT had a 26 per cent increased risk of breast cancer, a 29 per cent increased risk of heart disease and a 41 per cent chance of a stroke.[1] This was followed by the Million Women Study in 2003, which showed that an extra 20,000 cases of breast cancer had been caused by the use of HRT over a 10-year period, with 15,000 of those cases being linked to opposed HRT (oestrogen and progestogen), which is the combination most women use.[2]

There have been criticisms of the WHI study, saying that the wrong aged women were used and the wrong HRT preparation was given.[3] The Million Women Study has also been criticised for the questionnaire it used.[4]

But more recent studies have still shown that there is a higher risk of breast cancer when women take HRT (although there is less risk with just oestrogen on its own, which is given to women who have had a hysterectomy)[5] and also a higher risk of heart disease, strokes and clots.[6]

Even if the scientists can't agree about the degree of that risk, they do agree there is an increased risk, and as breast cancer is the most common cancer in the UK, having overtaken even lung cancer, which is mostly caused by smoking, I would not be prepared to take that risk. Figures from Cancer Research UK show that in 2006 more than 45,500 women in the UK were diagnosed with breast cancer (or around 125 women a day) and the incidence of breast cancer has increased by more than 50 per cent over the last 25 years. In the US, breast cancer is the second cause of cancer death because lung cancer is still the first. But the American Cancer Society notes that the US has the highest rates of breast cancer in the world.

The highest rates of breast cancer occur in Northern and West Europe and North America and the lowest rates are in Asia and in Eastern, Northern and Middle African countries. These statistics will become more relevant when we look at the dietary recommendations for the stages of the menopause (see chapters 7 and 14).

Every month or so there seems to be a new pronouncement on HRT and in March 2008 a panel of experts informed the public that the health risks had been greatly exaggerated and that HRT is safe to take for women aged between 50 and 59. It does not significantly raise heart disease risk and its impact on breast cancer is 'minimal' said a review from the first Global Summit on Menopause Related Issues. The experts also argued that although the risk of developing heart disease and breast cancer from HRT is slight it is dwarfed by other risks, such as obesity, drinking alcohol and eating fatty foods.

These findings are designed to set the record straight after years of health scares, which led many women to stop taking HRT, and the recommendation is to urge more doctors to prescribe HRT for women going through the menopause.

My initial reaction to this pronouncement was concern that many women may unnecessarily decide to take a drug with unpleasant side effects and serious health risks, believing it to be their only option. Apart from breast cancer and risk of heart disease there are many other potential side effects from HRT, including:

- endometrial (womb) cancer
- undesirable weight gain/loss
- breast tenderness/enlargement
- bloating
- depression
- thrombophlebitis (inflammation of a vein)
- elevated blood pressure
- reduced carbohydrate tolerance

- skin rashes
- hair loss
- abdominal cramps
- vaginal candidiasis (thrush)
- jaundice
- vomiting
- cystitis-like syndrome.

But the most significant pieces of research for me have been those that show the decline in breast cancer incidence since the publication of the WHI Study. First published in the *National Cancer Institute Bulletin* in 2007, researchers looked at breast cancer rates in the year following publication of the 2002 Women's Health Initiative Study. (Remember, this was a study whose results had either scared women off taking HRT and/or changed the prescribing habits of doctors.) These researchers found that the rate of breast cancer dropped by 12 per cent in 2003 among 50 to 69-year-old women, with 14,000 fewer women diagnosed in 2003. The researchers called this 'the largest single drop in breast cancer incidence within a single year'.

More reports since 2007 have linked the declining breast cancer rates to changes in HRT use. Follow-up data from the WHI of over 15,000 women showed that although the breast cancer rate was rising during the study, for those women who stopped HRT the number of breast cancers diagnosed fell by 28 per cent in just one year. Another WHI study on over 41,000 women showed a 50 per cent decrease in use of HRT between 2000 and 2003 with a subsequent decrease in the breast cancer rate of 43 per cent between 2002 and 2003.[7]

The researchers found that those women who decided to stay on HRT were at a far greater risk of breast cancer than they had previously thought. The chair of the WHI Executive Committee stated 'a woman who stayed on HRT for at least five years was found to double her risk of breast cancer' and 'this is very strong evidence that oestrogen plus progestin causes breast cancer'.[8] (Progestin is known as progestogen in the UK.)

The same effect has been seen in a study in the UK with a drop in HRT use and a parallel drop in breast cancer rates.[9] In a press release from Cancer Research UK, Dr David Parkin, the researcher of this study, was quoted as saying, 'We cannot be absolutely sure that the drop in both breast cancer rates and breast cancer risk is the direct result of women giving up HRT. But the parallel is striking and it will be interesting to see if this decline continues over the next few years.'

Although the breast cancer rate drops as the women stop HRT those women who take HRT have a 27 per cent higher breast cancer risk, even after three years of stopping taking HRT, compared to women who have never taken the drug.[10] The US National Institutes of Health funded the research and have stated that five years of combination (opposed) hormone therapy is harmful; meanwhile researchers at Cancer Research UK stress that women should only take HRT for as short a time as possible and only to treat the menopausal symptoms. The European Medicines Agency says that HRT should only be taken if the symptoms affect a woman's quality of life and should only be continued for as long as the benefits outweigh the risks.

In addition to the side effects given above, new research has shown that women on HRT have a 58 per cent higher risk of needing a knee joint replacement than women who have never taken it.[11]

BENEFITS OF TAKING HRT

Are there any benefits in taking HRT? Many women I have seen in the clinic have considered taking HRT because they think it will keep their skin and hair looking good and also give them more energy and a better sex drive. However, the research shows that there is no difference between women taking HRT and those taking a placebo in terms of quality of life, including getting better sleep, having more energy, feeling less depressed, experiencing sexual satisfaction or enjoying better general health.[12] This book can show you how you can use natural solutions to keep your skin and hair looking good and ensure you have enough energy and good moods.

HRT AND OSTEOPOROSIS

The WHI Study highlighted that HRT can protect against osteoporosis or fragile bones, showing that women on HRT had a 35 per cent reduction of osteoporotic fractures of the hip and 34 per cent for the spine.

However, because of the related risk of breast cancer and heart disease with HRT use, the European Medicines Agency has stated that HRT should not be used as a first-line treatment for osteoporosis in menopausal women.[13] This has also been confirmed by the Medicines and Healthcare Products Regulatory Body in 2007 (the UK equivalent of the FDA, or Food and Drug Administration, in the US), which says that HRT should only be used in the short term for the relief of menopausal symptoms and for postmenopausal women over 50, who are at increased risk of fracture. HRT should *only* be used to *prevent* osteoporosis if women are intolerant of, or contraindicated for, other osteoporosis drugs. In a nutshell, HRT is not recommended as a 'catch all' to prevent osteoporosis.

It is also worth bearing in mind with HRT that as soon as the drug is stopped any benefits to your bones are lost.[14] If you did decide to take HRT primarily for your bone health you would have to take it for the rest of your life, when, at present, it is recommended that women only take HRT for a maximum of five years for the menopausal symptoms, which usually happen around the age of 50. The risk of fractures is greatest around the age of 75, so there really is no point in taking HRT thinking it is going to help your bones.

HRT AND OTHER HEALTH CONDITIONS

It was also thought previously that HRT could help prevent dementia, memory loss and Alzheimer's but the US FDA make it clear that HRT has never been approved for these problems and, in fact, research has now shown that HRT can actually increase the risk of developing dementia.[15]

The same is unfortunately true for urinary incontinence, as it has been found that HRT can also increase the severity of the problem.[16]

There are so many natural solutions that can help ease the menopausal symptoms and reduce health risks such as osteoporosis and heart disease that I believe it is not worth taking HRT for the maximum recommended period of five years.

BIOIDENTICAL HORMONES

This is the hot potato of both the conventional and nutritional medicine world. Bioidentical hormone replacement has been used in the US for many years but interest has been sparked recently around the world by media interest in this topic. I will look at bioidentical hormones in some detail in this section, because many doctors are now prescribing these for women in the UK and some women are even buying them independently from the internet.

WHAT ARE BIOIDENTICAL HORMONES?

Bioidentical hormones are chemically similar in structure to the hormones your body would produce naturally, so they could include oestradiol, oestriol, testosterone and progesterone, DHEA (a steroid hormone that declines with age), pregnenolone and human growth hormone. They are considered to be more 'natural' than the synthetic versions used in many HRT drugs. In the US they are often connected to individualised hormone therapy treatment because practitioners use compounding pharmacies that will make up different prescriptions of these bioidentical hormones, often based on the results of saliva or blood tests. It is this 'tailoring' of bioidentical hormones for an individual patient that makes them different and, in many people's eyes, more 'natural' and therefore better.

But to be clear from the outset, these hormones are still made in a lab in the same way that conventional HRT would be made and from the same sources. If asked whether I would consider bioidentical hormones a 'natural solution' I would have to say no, for a number of reasons.

Firstly, these are hormones just as in HRT except that they are marketed as having a molecular structure similar to our own. But, there are conventional HRT preparations that contain bioidentical hormones; they are just not tailored individually based on hormone testing. No matter what stage of the menopause you are at, by replacing hormones that are naturally decreasing, you are basically telling your body that its natural rhythm is 'wrong' and that this decline should not be happening.

Secondly, when would you stop taking them? If it were indeed correct to replace these naturally declining hormones then you would need to take them for ever. And indeed, some women do think it is fine to take these hormones indefinitely.

Thirdly, these are still hormones and I believe they should be on prescription like any drug. Adding back these hormones requires a judgement as to which hormone you need and in what dose or combination with other hormones. Hormone levels would still need to be adjusted as you go through the different stages of the menopause because of their individual nature.

ARE BIOIDENTICAL HORMONES SAFER THAN HRT?

If you have decided, for whatever reason, that you are going to take HRT, is it safer to take these bioidentical hormones than conventional HRT? Bioidentical hormone replacement therapy has been promoted as being safer, more natural and more effective than conventional HRT but there is a lack of scientific evidence to support these claims. For instance, as oestriol is a 'weaker' oestrogen than oestradiol it could be assumed that it may carry a lesser risk of breast cancer but there are no randomised controlled trials to show this. Some researchers argue that, in general, bioidentical hormones are safer in terms of breast cancer and heart disease than conventional HRT,[17] but other research reports there is no evidence to show that they are safer.[18] I believe you are still adding back hormones (bioidentical or not) during a stage in your life when they are naturally decreasing and this is where the risk is found.

A number of associations in the UK and US have stated that bioidentical hormones carry the same risks and benefits as non-bioidentical hormones.[19] Bioidentical hormones are not regulated in the UK or by the FDA in America, which has sent out warning letters to pharmacies in the US about using claims of safety and effectiveness of bioidentical hormones to market them.

This means that if you are taking bioidentical hormones in the UK you are taking an unlicensed drug. Although they are promoted as being tailored and individualised to your own hormone profiles, it has become apparent from patients I have seen who have been put on these hormones that many UK doctors recommending them are not basing the dosages or choice of hormones on any kind of hormone testing. For example, if a woman feels tired or has a lack of sex drive then testosterone is added, without any test to confirm the need for it.

It has also become obvious from patients I have seen that no testing has been done after they have been on the hormones for a couple of months. I suggested to one patient who had come for nutritional advice that she have a hormone test, considering that she had been on bioidentical hormones for a few months. The results showed that she had extremely high testosterone levels, which over time could have caused excess facial hair growth, acne, deepening of the voice and aggressive behaviour.

Some women are taking up to eight hormones together (see page 182), either in a cream applied to the skin or in lozenges placed in the cheek or under the tongue. There is no scientific agreement on the dosages, combinations and length of time that you use these bioidentical hormones. Try not to get sucked in by the hype and the celebrity endorsements. These are not natural products, they are drugs and they are unlicensed.

In Australia a number of cases of womb cancer from using bioidentical hormones have been noted. This can occur if the ratio of oestrogen to progesterone is not correct, which can cause too much build up of the womb lining, leading to a risk of endometrial (womb) cancer.[20] So if you *are* taking these hormones ensure you have regular ultrasound scans to monitor your endometrium (womb lining).

BIOIDENTICAL HORMONES AND PREMATURE MENOPAUSE

I would not recommend either conventional or bioidentical HRT to any women going through the menopause. Again, the exception to this is if you need HRT because you have gone through a premature menopause (premature ovarian failure) before the age of 40 (see page 115). In such a situation you are really replacing those hormones that should naturally be circulating in your body. If you can do that with more 'natural' hormones, then biodentical hormones would seem a better choice because you are replacing those hormones in the same molecular form that your own body would have produced them rather than a synthetic version.

Some bioidentical hormones are available on prescription in the UK. These include Hormonin (containing oestradiol, oestrone and oestrial) and different brands of vaginal oestrogen. The vaginal ones that contain oestradiol are the most carcinogenic but there are some that contain oestriol, a less potent form of oestrogen (such as Ovestin and Ortho-Gynest), so ask your doctor about them rather than trying to self-prescribe via the internet. Micronised progesterone (see below) known as Utrogestan is also available on prescription in the UK now.

Make sure you are properly monitored at all times, and that progesterone levels are sufficient to prevent the endometrium (womb lining) from building up abnormally.

ORDERING DRUGS FROM THE INTERNET

Never try to self-prescribe your own drugs via the internet, even if they seem readily available. It is very important to seek the advice of a professional to ensure you do not cause yourself any harm.

Progesterone as a bioidentical hormone

I would like to discuss the use of progesterone here because this bioidentical hormone is more widely used than any of the others and is freely available on the internet, usually in the form of a topical cream. Again, it is often marketed as 'natural' progesterone cream because it is synthesised in the lab from wild yam and is chemically identical to the progesterone produced by your body. Synthetic progesterones are known as 'progestogens' or 'progestins' in the US, and are used in many conventional HRTs and also in the Pill. In conventional HRT, progestogens can be derived from progesterone and these are known as dydrogesterone and medroxyprogesterone; it can also be derived from testosterone (known as norethisterone).

Progesterone, when taken by mouth, is broken down too much by the liver, which means that not enough ends up in the bloodstream (there is not the same problem with progestogens). To get round this, progesterone is often used as a cream, which is absorbed through the skin, thus bypassing the liver, or in a micronised form where it is broken down into tiny particles to aid absorption.

186

The common perception is that oestrogen is the 'bad' hormone and progesterone is the 'good' hormone, but they both play important roles in the body. We all think of oestrogen as being the culprit in terms of breast cancer, but in fact progesterone can also increase the risk of breast cancer. There are progesterone receptor positive breast cancers as well as oestrogen receptor positive ones. In fact, up to 65 per cent of oestrogen receptor positive breast cancers are also progesterone receptor positive. We know that progesterone promotes angiogenesis,[21] where new blood vessels form tumours and the blood supply keeps them growing; progesterone also promotes cell proliferation.[22] Progesterone receptors can also be involved in 'turning on' breast cancer cell growth.

So what about the supposed benefits of using progesterone? Recent research has shown that using progesterone cream does not have any beneficial effect on bone density and is no different to a placebo over a three-year period.[23] Additionally, it does not show any benefit versus a placebo in relieving the symptoms of the menopause such as hot flushes and night sweats but actually increases the risk of headaches.[24]

MY TAKE ON BIOIDENTICAL HORMONES

My advice, unless you are going through an early menopause, is to steer clear of bioidentical hormones – do not be fooled into thinking you are using 'natural' remedies. You are still using hormone replacement therapy; it is just that the molecular structure of bioidentical hormones is more similar to what your body produces. Furthermore, you should not be lulled into thinking that because these bioidentical hormones are made from natural sources they are 'better' than conventional HRT. Yes, they are made from soya and yam in the laboratory, but so are many of the conventional HRTs and there is no soya or yam left in the end product of either.

For me, the most important issue with regard to HRT or bioidentical hormones is that adding any form of synthetic or 'natural' hormones to your body does not permit it to go through the transition of the menopause and out the other side in a natural way.

I believe that by using natural solutions – which included adopting a healthy, hormone-balancing diet with appropriate vitamins and minerals, taking useful herbs and making lifestyle changes – you are giving your body the tools it needs to find the hormonal balance that is appropriate for the stage of the menopause you are experiencing. Using these natural methods, you are not taking a drug that can expose you to the risk of serious health problems such as breast cancer, heart disease or stroke.

Q&A

If I do decide to go on HRT what would be the best way to take it?
First you should try the natural solutions outlined in this book for this natural period of change in your life. But if you want to take HRT then you have a number of choices.

You could take bioidentical hormones because even though it is not known whether they are safer than conventional HRT, at least they may be easier for your body to utilise as they are chemically identical to what you naturally produce. You can ask your doctor for these, as they are available on prescription as Hormonin (containing oestradiol, oestrone and oestrial) and Utrogestan (micronised progesterone), or you could see a private doctor who specialises in bioidentical hormones.

The primary concern is to manage the symptoms and to use the lowest dose possible to achieve that. I believe it is better not to individualise the hormones on the basis of blood or salivary tests, as there is no agreement on what the levels should be during the menopause. But I recommend you have tests about three months after taking the hormones to make sure that your levels are not too high.

If you decide to use conventional HRT then you have a choice about how you take it. You could use an oestrogen patch and take micronised progesterone by mouth, or you could have a combined patch. It is better to use patches or gel to deliver the oestrogen as the hormone is delivered through the skin. When oestrogen is taken by mouth, a large part of the hormone is lost as it is broken down by your liver, so you have to start off with a larger dose to get enough in the bloodstream.

Where possible, if you are using a synthetic progesterone (progestogen), get it in the form of dydrogesterone or medroxy-progesterone, which are derived from progesterone rather than from norethisterone, a derivative of testosterone. Dydrogesterone and medroxyprogesterone originate from the hormone you are aiming to replace but norethisterone and others are derived from testosterone, which can have side effects such as mood swings and growth of facial hair.

I have been on HRT for nearly six years now and I would like to come off it. What is the best way to do this?
The question I am asked most often is 'Should I just suddenly stop HRT or should I come off it gradually?' You should talk to your doctor about your decision to come off HRT and have any check-ups that might be needed. My recommendation is always that a gradual weaning process is easier on your body. Stopping HRT suddenly is similar to going 'cold turkey' and there have been reports of 'rebound' effects from the quick withdrawal of the hormones. The rebound effects can actually give tremendous hot flushes and seemingly worsened menopausal symptoms.

I suggest that you take three months to wean yourself off HRT gradually. First, put into place the nutritional recommendations in

Part One of this book so that you are in the best of health by the time you stop HRT. Ask your doctor for a lower dose and if you cannot reduce the dose of the HRT, you could switch to a patch. Because the patch delivers oestrogen through the skin and does not have to be broken down by the liver first, you can get by with a lower dose than if it is taken orally. If you take a combined HRT do not alter the dose of the progestogen (or progesterone) as that part of the drug protects your endometrium (womb lining) from building up abnormally, as discussed above.

As a rule, you would not take herbs and HRT together but as you wean yourself off the HRT over the three months, you could use herbs (see page 140) to cushion the withdrawal effects.

CHAPTER 12

TESTS AND SCANS

In this chapter you will find information about tests and scans you can have that are particularly useful around the time of the menopause when your body changes and opens you up to higher risk for certain conditions. This is the 'know where you stand section', to help you find out about certain aspects of your health and make decisions about what action you may or may not need to take.

There are a number of tests your doctor might suggest as you go through this stage of your life, and there are some nutritional tests which I think are extremely useful to have as they give different information to the standard medical ones.

PRIVATE CT SCANS

Although I think that testing can be very helpful I do have concerns about private CT scans either for scanning the whole body or specific parts such as colon, heart or lungs. Normally CT scans are used when somebody is thought to be at risk of a particular disease but there is now a growing trend for healthy people to opt for private CT scans.

CT scans pass X-rays through sections of a person's body and the imaging system produces slices of those areas. These slices are then reconstructed using a computer to produce images of tissue and internal organs.

My concern is that the scan itself can deliver the equivalent of between 500 and 1,000 chest X-rays. If somebody is worried about having cancer then the technique, the CT scan, used to investigate the problem can be delivering levels of radiation that could trigger cell mutation. The Committee on the Medical Aspects of Radiation in the Environment (Comare) states that one in 50 people who are scanned every five years, from the age of 40 onwards, could die from a malignancy caused by the repeated radiation exposure. Research from the US is suggesting that radiation exposure from these types of scans could make up 2 per cent of cancers.

The scan could also pick up conditions that are not medically significant but could lead to further invasive investigations and cause needless anxiety.

The US FDA has issued a publication called 'Full body CT scans – What you need to know' (www.fda.gov) stating that there are no proven benefits of scans for healthy people. The idea of taking preventative action, finding unsuspected disease and uncovering problems while they are treatable all sounds great, almost too good to be true! However, at this time the Food and Drug Administration (FDA) knows of no scientific evidence demonstrating that whole-body scanning of individuals without symptoms provides more benefit than harm to people being screened.

With any procedure you should always weigh up the risks versus the benefits and I think that this type of scanning could actually do more harm than good. Think carefully before paying for one of these scans, which are expensive and may cause more worry than they are promoted to alleviate.

BONE DENSITY SCAN

It is important to know your bone health at the earliest age possible. Fracture risk is greatest in our seventies to eighties but if you wait until you are in your seventies to find out whether you have a major problem it may be too late to help yourself. Knowing early about poor bone health means you can take active steps to do something about it.

Osteoporosis is preventable but silent so you would not know you had a problem until you maybe fractured a bone, just by stubbing your toe lightly for example. (For more detailed information on osteoporosis see chapter 15.)

As we reach our peak bone density around the age of 25 to 30, the ideal scenario would be to have a bone scan in our thirties and we would then have a baseline to compare with when we got to the menopause.

According to the UK's National Osteoporosis Society, one in two women over the age of 50 will get osteoporosis. This is compared to one in nine for breast cancer and yet we have a national screening programme for breast cancer in the UK and nothing for osteoporosis. In fact, osteoporosis is a bigger killer than ovarian, cervical and womb cancers combined. Have a look at page 209 to see the risk factors for osteoporosis. If you have any of the risk factors I recommend you have a scan even if you have to pay for it privately. A scan is the best way to check your bone health and the earlier you know if you have a problem then the more you can do to prevent it becoming worse. The best way to check on your bone health is to have a scan. There are a number of different scans available which I have listed below.

DEXA SCAN (DUAL ENERGY X-RAY ABSORPTIOMETRY)

This is considered to be the best way to assess osteoporotic risk. It is different from an ordinary X-ray machine in that it passes two X-ray beams (one low and one high energy), usually through the hip and spine, and the DEXA scanner can calculate the bone density by the difference between the two beams. The amount of X-ray is equivalent to about one chest X-ray.

The World Health Organisation (WHO) defines osteoporosis by a measurement called a T score and it is scored as:

Normal: T score = above -1.0
Osteopenia (low bone density): T score = between -1.0 and -2.5
Osteoporosis: T score = less than -2.5

CT SCAN

CT scanning is not routinely used for assessing osteoporosis risk because it is very expensive and also delivers a much higher level of radiation than the DEXA scan.

QUANTITATIVE ULTRASOUND SCANS (QUS)

With QUS, sound waves are passed through the heel of the foot, which reflects the same type of trabecular bone as in the hip. Like the DEXA machines, QUS machines give a T score but they assess the quality of the bone (elasticity and stiffness) rather than density.

QUS are valuable because the scan is inexpensive and avoids the use of X-rays. I use a QUS machine in my clinic and would only suggest you to go on to have a DEXA scan if your reading from the QUS came up low.

Research has looked at giving perimenopausal women bone scans (DEXA and QUS) to see whether it is possible to predict future fractures.[1] It has been shown that scanning women in the lead-up to the menopause can help predict fractures up to 10 years later, with QUS being a better predictor of future fractures than DEXA scanning.

BONE TURNOVER TEST

You may have been told that your bone density is low (osteopenic), and have decided to increase your exercise and follow the dietary and supplement recommendations in this book. How would you know that they are working? The same applies if you are prescribed a drug for osteoporosis. A follow-up scan would not usually be offered until two years later, which is quite a long time to wait to know that what you have done or taken has made a difference. This is where the measurement of bone turnover comes in.

In your urine, you excrete biochemical markers, which show how fast or slowly your bone is breaking down. The higher the levels of these markers in the urine, the faster you are losing bone, so measuring bone turnover can be a useful way of monitoring treatment. The best approach is to have a scan and then if the bone density isn't as good as it should be to have a bone turnover test as soon as possible. You would then need to put changes in place to improve your bone health and in three months' time you should retest the bone turnover. The results from that follow-up bone turnover test should then be lower if what you are doing is working. If the turnover results are not lower then you need to rethink what you are taking or doing because it is not affecting the loss of bone.

It is acknowledged that measuring bone mineral density using DEXA does not capture all the risk factors for osteoporosis so having the extra benefit of a bone turnover test is really helpful.

Research has shown that in postmenopausal women osteoporosis levels of bone resorption markers above the upper limit of the range are associated with an increased risk of hip, vertebral (spinal) and non-vertebral fractures, independent of bone mineral density.[2]

Markers of bone turnover can also be used to predict the rate of bone loss in postmenopausal women and to assess the risk of fractures. Research suggests that markers of bone turnover appear to be even more strongly associated with fracture risk than bone mineral density.[3] (This test can be organised by post, see Useful Resources on page 283.)

OTHER USEFUL TESTS

In chapter 17 I cover other tests that are useful after the menopause. These same tests can also be helpful during the perimenopause, as being forewarned can mean you are forearmed and can take action to stop the problem becoming worse.

PART THREE

A NEW BEGINNING BEYOND THE MENOPAUSE

CHAPTER 13

THROUGH THE MENOPAUSE

On average, women spend around five years going through the menopause (the perimenopause) before reaching the point of 'menopause', your last ever period, and then entering the postmenopausal stage. You are classed as being postmenopausal once you have had one year with no periods.

Beyond the menopause you can now expect to live anywhere between 30 and 50 years in this stage of your life – a good long while! With such a promising stretch of time ahead of you it is good to know what you can do to keep yourself healthy both physically and mentally.

Much has been written about the menopause but many women have said to me that there is very little written about what women should be doing to look after themselves in this postmenopausal stage. So in some ways this is one of the most important parts of the book and the information in this section can help you not only have a good quantity of years but, I think more importantly, a good quality of years.

I will cover the best nutritional advice for this stage in your life as well as the most important supplements that you should take and address key health issues that are likely to affect you. I will also list further tests that I consider important to have done.

CAN I TEST TO SEE IF I AM POSTMENOPAUSAL?

If you have not had a period for at least a year then a blood test would be accurate in showing whether you are postmenopausal. Before then, as described on page 119, levels of FSH (follicle stimulating hormone) could be fluctuating, which means that a test would not be such a reliable indicator. However, at this postmenopausal stage a blood test would show high FSH levels and low oestrogen (oestradiol) and can provide a clear answer for you.

COULD I STILL GET PREGNANT BEYOND THE MENOPAUSE?

The rule of thumb is that you are contraceptively safe if you are over 50 and have had one year free of periods. If the menopause has happened before the age of 50 then you should give yourself two years to be absolutely sure.

SKIN, HAIR AND NAILS

You would be forgiven for thinking that your skin and hair are going to get duller and drier, and your nails more brittle, purely due to the menopause; this is a common misconception. In fact, there will be changes anyway because you are getting older so they may not be caused by the menopause. For whatever reason they occur, by using natural remedies suggested in the following section you can keep yourself looking and feeling good.

CHAPTER 14

YOUR DIET, FOOD SUPPLEMENTS AND EXERCISE

YOUR DIET

You should continue to follow my Twelve-Step Hormone Balancing Diet on page 18 and although your hormones will be fairly stable now, it will help you to keep yourself healthy, particularly your heart and bones.

Always keep in your mind to 'eat a rainbow' and that way you will be getting a wide selection of antioxidants from fruit and vegetables, which are not only beneficial for anti-ageing but also for your heart and bone health. Pay particular attention to the essential fatty acids found in oily fish, nuts and seeds, as these will help control inflammation that can affect not only your joints and risk of osteoporosis but also your heart (see section on Inflammation on page 231) and can help to control cholesterol.

A good intake of fruit and vegetables will keep your body more alkaline, which is good for your bones, and the consumption of fruits and vegetables, particularly green leafy vegetables and vitamin C-rich fruits and vegetables, seems to have a protective effect against coronary heart disease.[1] You will also be getting vitamin K from the green vegetables and because vitamin K is a fat-soluble vitamin you can increase its absorption by drizzling on some oil, such as flaxseed (linseed) oil, on your vegetables after cooking.

If you suffer from high blood pressure a good intake of fruit and vegetables is very important. In America a diet called DASH (dietary approaches to stop hypertension/high blood pressure) has been launched, which has been shown to be as good as or even better than the effects of drugs. It is now being suggested as a first-line treatment for high blood pressure as it has been shown to lower moderately high blood pressure in 14 days (see www.nhibi.nih.gov). Meat is thought to be one of the main culprits in raising high blood pressure, mainly because it creates an inflammatory effect, so it is suggested that this is substituted with fish and an increase in fruit and vegetables. The DASH diet also limits refined carbohydrates such as sugar and products made with white flour such as biscuits, bread and cakes. It also reduces saturated fats and salt.

We should all avoid too much salt in our diets but this is of particular importance if you have high blood pressure. Salt is often used as a preservative and is added to most processed, pre-packaged foods. It is often used in low-fat foods in order to improve the taste. If you are using salt, only use it in cooking and never add it to your food at the table. As you reduce the salt you use, your tastebuds adjust and you can learn to appreciate the more subtle flavours that were once hidden.

Many foods today claim to be 'reduced salt' or 'low salt' but this can be confusing when labels talk of sodium. To find out how much salt is in a food, multiply the sodium content on the label by 2.5. You should aim for less than 5g of salt a day.

When using salt choose sea salt or rock salt rather than the usual table salt (which can contain chemicals to make it flow), or you could consider using tamari (wheat-free soy sauce) and miso (soya paste) to give an alternative salty taste. You can also try some of these other suggestions below instead of salt:

- basil
- bay leaf
- chives
- cinnamon
- cloves
- cumin
- curry powder
- dill
- garlic
- ginger
- lemon
- marjoram
- paprika
- parsley
- rosemary
- sage.

You should still keep your blood sugar under control by eating little and often as this will not only keep mood swings at bay but also can help to control your weight and control inflammation.

Unfortunately, your metabolism slows down as you get older so it means that you need to eat healthily to keep your weight under control. If you need extra help with this then see chapter 10. It is important for your heart health, prevention of diabetes and also blood pressure to keep your weight under control. According to the British Heart Foundation, reducing your weight by as little as 11lb (5kg) can reduce blood pressure in most people who are more than 10 per cent over the ideal weight.

Your metabolism is also governed by how much muscle you have so this is covered in the Exercise section below.

For your bone health, you should keep your diet more alkaline (see page 210) and less acidic in order to keep calcium in your skeleton. (See the Appendix, page 279, for a list of non-dairy foods and their calcium content which shows that you can get calcium from a good range of foods and not just dairy.) If you want to have dairy foods, concentrate on live plain organic yogurt as the friendly bacteria will help to control inflammation.

Make sure you are drinking enough fluids, which can be in the form of plain water and herbal teas. Be careful of caffeine as this can increase problems with inflammation because it is a stimulant. You also need to keep alcohol to a minimum because it can increase the risk of heart disease, high blood pressure, cancer and stroke. Keep to a maximum of two units on any one day and try to have days off in the week so you are not drinking every night.

SMOKING

When talking about your long-term health in the postmenopause, I have to include smoking. If you haven't stopped yet, this is the time. By giving up smoking you reduce your risk of heart attacks (it damages the heart muscle), high blood pressure (because it constricts your arteries), stroke and osteoporosis. Smoking also ages you faster.

You should still eat phytoestrogens because they are good for your general health as well as your heart and bone health. Research has shown that a daily intake of soya (about 3½fl oz/100ml soya milk or the equivalent) reduces the risk of hip fractures by 20–30 per cent.[2] Don't just focus on soya; have a good variety of all the legumes including chickpeas, kidney beans and lentils.

SUPPLEMENTS

During this stage in your life you want a good maintenance supplement programme to keep you healthy. It needs to give you the energy for a good quality of life and at the same time give you the right nutrients that help to work on disease prevention. There may also be certain nutrients that you will have to add in for a short while, usually around three months if you have to correct a problem, and carry on with the maintenance programme after that.

I am assuming that you are eating well because supplements are not a substitute for a healthy diet. I am going to outline a good maintenance programme of supplements that I think all women at this stage in their life should take.

YOUR MAINTENANCE SUPPLEMENT PROGRAMME

Your daily programme should include:

- multivitamin and mineral
- Omega 3 fish oils (with 770mg EPA and 510mg DHA)
- vitamin C (500mg twice a day).

Multivitamin and mineral

This is the foundation of your supplement programme and should be a multivitamin and mineral that is designed for use at this stage in your life, rather than just a general multi for a man or woman of any age. You want it to contain good levels of antioxidants (vitamins A, E, zinc and selenium) for your heart and bone health and for their anti-ageing effects. Vitamin E has extra benefits for your heart health as shown in one study where patients with arteriosclerosis were either given vitamin E or a placebo. Vitamin E reduced the risk of a heart attack by 75 per cent[3] as it helps to prevent abnormal blood clotting.

Good levels of the B vitamins are important because they are not only good for energy and are your 'stress' vitamins but they also help to control homocysteine (especially B6, B12 and folic acid). In one study those people who had high homocysteine levels (over 14mmol/L) had approximately 70 per cent higher hip fracture risk than those with lower levels.[4]

The multi should also contain good levels of calcium, magnesium, boron and vitamin D for your bone health and the calcium should be in the form of citrate and the vitamin D as D3. Vitamin D is now known to be helpful not only for the prevention of osteoporosis but also plays a part in preventing heart disease, cancer and slowing down the ageing process. The calcium and magnesium can also be helpful if you have high blood pressure.

(The multivitamin and mineral I use in the clinic is called Meno Plus and is available from www.naturalhealthpractice.com. It also contains digestive enzymes for improved absorption.)

Omega 3 fish oils

Omega 3 fish oils, containing both EPA (eicosapentaenoic acid) and DHA (docosahexenoic acid) are very important to take in supplement form as they have a beneficial anti-inflammatory effect on your body. This anti-inflammatory effect will benefit your heart, brain, bones and joints. The other bonus is that by controlling inflammation you are controlling the ageing process from the inside out.

We also know that those people with higher levels of Omega 3 fats in their body have less periodontal disease. Periodontal disease is another manifestation of chronic inflammation and there can be increased bone loss in the jaw as well as gingivitis, and what happens in the mouth and jaw can also be a reflection of what is happening in the rest of your skeleton. However, don't supplement with Omega 6 (such as evening primrose oil), as those with higher levels of Omega 6 oils are found to have more periodontal disease.[5] The Omega 6 oils, as mentioned on page 29, can create more inflammation, and there is generally too much Omega 6 in the body and not enough Omega 3.

A study published in 2009 showed that Omega 3 oils help to prevent blood clotting and lower blood pressure.[6] This is why it is even more crucial to take Omega 3 if you know you already have heart disease.

The DHA in the fish oils can also help reduce the formation of plaque in the brain, helping your brain to function well as you get older and protect against age-related macular degeneration (see page 253).

The most staggering piece of information came out in 2009 from the Harvard School of Public Health, which stated that Omega 3 deficient diets cause up to 96,000 preventable deaths a year in the US.[7] The researchers estimated the number of deaths resulting from 12 preventable causes and Omega 3 deficiency ranked as the sixth highest killer of Americans. A deficiency in these fats was classed as a bigger killer than high intake of trans fats. (If you want to know if you are deficient in Omega 3 fatty acids see Useful Resources on page 283 for a test you can do by post.)

Vitamin C

There will never be enough vitamin C in a multi so you need to take this separately. Vitamin C is an important antioxidant and is also beneficial for your immune function. Vitamin C is especially important at this time in your life because it is crucial for the manufacture of collagen, which is important for your bone health as it makes up 90 per cent of your bone matrix, gives your skin its elasticity and keeps your blood vessels strong to prevent easy bruising. It is also essential for joints, muscles, ligaments and tendons. Research has shown that those older people who have higher total or supplemental intake of vitamin C have fewer hip fractures than people with the lowest intakes.[8]

Choose vitamin C in the alkaline form, magnesium ascorbate, as this is going to be gentler on your digestive system than the more common acidic form as ascorbic acid.

EXERCISE

Exercise is important not only for prevention of osteoporosis but also for your heart health so its importance beyond the menopause cannot be over-stressed. Refer back to chapters 3 and 9 for advice on how and when to exercise. Regular exercise has been shown to increase joint mobility and flexibility in arthritis suffers. It can also help keep your weight down as being overweight puts extra pressure on bones and joints.

Aim to take regular aerobic exercise for 30 to 40 minutes, three times a week, as it has been shown to lower blood pressure and prevent heart attacks. Exercise is also another way of lowering inflammation, which is a factor in so many age-related diseases.[9]

Keeping active can also help to increase your life span and protect against Alzheimer's. Research at the University of California at Stanford, reported in the journal *Archives of Internal Medicine*, compared members of a running club and healthy non-running individuals all over the age of 50 at the start of the study. Twice as many non-runners had died than runners after 19 years. The researchers believe that running may not just boost health and improve immunity but also increase cognitive performance. This is supported by a study undertaken at the University of Kansas School of Medicine, reported in *Neurology*, which concluded that by exercising, individuals with early Alzheimer's may have better cognitive performance through increased blood flow to the head. Poor blood flow to the head can result in loss of memory.

Another study from scientists at the University of Calgary in Canada also proved that regular physical activity benefits blood flow to the brain, which in turn helps mental agility. The researchers compared two groups of women with the average age of 65. One group took part in regular exercise while the other was inactive. Their blood flow, heart health and brain power were then tested. Not only did the active group have lower blood pressure and better blood flow, they also scored higher in mental agility tests proving that basic fitness – something as simple as walking every day – is critical to staying mentally sharp as we age.

As well as aerobic exercise you want to include exercises that improve your balance such as yoga because the more co-ordinated you are the less chance you have of falling over and then breaking a bone. You should also include exercises to improve your strength because both balance and strength can help prevent falls and fractures.[10]

Strength training such as weight resistance is a good way of both maintaining your muscle tone and improving balance. Unfortunately as we get older we lose muscle due to the drop in oestrogen. Muscle is metabolically active so the more muscle you have the more fat you burn and, because your muscles are attached to the ends of your bones, as you strengthen the muscles you also strengthen your bones.

CHAPTER 15

OSTEOPOROSIS – HOW TO PREVENT, STOP AND EVEN REVERSE IT

One of the biggest risks for women past the menopause is osteoporosis. If you have not had a bone density scan already, then arrange to have one as soon as you can so you know where you currently stand, and if your bone density is low then do a bone turnover test to see whether you are actively losing bone on a daily basis. (For more on tests and scans see chapter 12.)

RISK FACTORS FOR OSTEOPOROSIS

There are a number of risk factors for osteoporosis that apply no matter what your age. It is worth thinking about whether you might be more at risk, in which case the tests and scans recommended above become even more important. You would also be well advised to place more emphasis on dietary recommendations than a woman who does not have an increased risk.

You are at risk of osteoporosis if you say 'Yes' to any of the following statements.

- You have a family history of osteoporosis.
- Your periods stopped for over six months when you were younger.
- You had anorexia.
- You went through the menopause before the age of 45, either naturally occurring or because of surgery or chemotherapy.
- You have been or are a smoker.
- You have taken medications such as steroids, heparin, anti-convulsants, diuretics, long-term laxatives or antacids.
- You are inactive.
- You got shorter with age.
- You have a slim frame.
- You have digestive problems such as Crohn's or coeliac.
- You drink more than seven units of alcohol a week.
- You have more than two cups of coffee or regular tea per day.

YOUR DIET AND SUPPLEMENTS

The emphasis for preventing and treating osteoporosis is to make your diet more alkaline. Research on the rate of hip fractures in women around the world has shown that the more acidic the diet becomes the higher the risk of hip fractures. Calcium neutralises acid so the more acidic your food the more calcium has to be taken out of your bones to make the body more alkaline again.

The most acid-producing foods are animal protein and the chart opposite[1] shows the difference in rate of hip fractures depending on the amount of animal protein in the diet. As the animal protein intake increases so does the risk of hip fracture.

Country	Hip fractures per 100,000 person years	Animal protein (grams per day)	Vegetable protein (grams per day)
Nigeria	0.8	8.1	40.2
China	2.9	10.7	51.2
UK	116.5	54.4	36.6
US	120.3	70.1	32.9

The more fruit and vegetables you eat the more alkaline your body becomes and there will be less loss of calcium from your bones. You do need to eat some protein though, so choose good quality animal protein such as eggs and fish and also include vegetable protein, then make sure that you are having good amounts of alkaline fruit and vegetables.

Your skeleton acts like a buffer and the more acidic your diet becomes the more calcium you will lose to neutralise that acid, and the reverse is true when you make the body more alkaline. The power of fruit and vegetables to keep your bones healthy is enormous. Indeed, one study described fruit and vegetables as 'the unexpected natural answer to the question of osteoporosis prevention'.[2]

Research has shown that higher intakes of animal protein are associated with lower bone density whereas higher intakes of vegetable protein are linked with better bone density[3] and a seven-year study of older women showed that those who consumed a high animal protein diet had more bone loss and a greater risk of hip fractures than women with a lower animal protein intake.[4]

Another point to bear in mind is that cheese, a traditional source of calcium, is one of the most acidic foods you can eat and you can actually be losing more calcium from your bones than the amount of calcium you will get from the cheese.[5]

OTHER FOODS AND DRINKS TO REDUCE OR ELIMINATE

Caffeine, sugar and alcohol

Both coffee and sugar cause an acidic reaction similar to that triggered by animal protein and have the same effect of leaching calcium from your bones.

Tea also contains caffeine, although not as much as coffee, so the acidic effect is reduced. However, if you like your cuppa, take care not to drink it at mealtimes because the tannin in tea binds to important minerals such as calcium and zinc and prevents their absorption in the digestive tract. Leave a gap of at least half-an-hour before or after eating if you are going to have a cup of regular black tea.

Alcohol also contributes to osteoporosis because it acts as a diuretic, leaching out valuable minerals such as calcium and magnesium. This increases bone loss and the incidence of fractures.

Bran

Bran is a refined food that contains substances called 'phytates'. These act like a magnet, attracting valuable minerals such as calcium and zinc and magnesium, which are essential for your bones and general health. These minerals bind to the phytates and are then excreted, along with the bran, from the digestive tract, so don't add refined bran to your cereals. It is better to eat bran in the form that nature intended, as part of the whole grain (such as brown rice or oats).

Spinach and rhubarb

Both spinach and rhubarb contain oxalic acid, which reacts with calcium in the digestive system and stops it being absorbed, so if you have osteoporosis they should be avoided and you should reduce your intake if you are worried about your bone health.

Fizzy soft drinks

Phosphoric acid is added to fizzy soft drinks to give a tangy taste and higher levels of phosphorus in the blood tell your body to release calcium from the bones to balance out the phosphorus. Recent research has shown that drinking just four colas a week is associated with lower bone density.[6]

MEASURING THE ACIDITY AND ALKALINITY OF YOUR DIET

Your ideal diet would be one where 70 to 80 per cent of your food is alkaline and 20 to 30 per cent is acid. But how can you tell if you are achieving this?

Acid and alkaline is measured as pH on a scale of 0 to 14 with a pH of 7 being neutral. Anything below 7 is acid and anything above 7 is alkaline (also called base). Testing your blood pH will not help as your body keeps the pH of your blood between 7.35–7.45 and if it goes outside that range either way you would become ill.

Research has looked at whether testing the pH of urine could be a useful indicator of whether a person is eating the right balance of acid and alkaline foods. A study of people between the ages of 39 and 78 in the UK showed that a higher fruit and vegetable intake and lower consumption of meat was significantly associated with a more alkaline urine pH.[7] The normal range for the pH of urine is 4.5–8.4 but the more ideal alkaline range would be 6.5–7.5. You can buy urine dip sticks for testing pH.

Testing saliva for pH is not recommended as this will reflect what you have just put in your mouth, whereas with urine you are measuring the result of the breakdown of the food and drink you have eaten.

CONTROL INFLAMMATION

We have seen how controlling inflammation is important in relation to heart disease but it is also relevant to osteoporosis as we know that inflammation can lead to increased bone breakdown,[8] so put into place the dietary and supplement recommendations (see page 200) to help control it. Pay particular attention to the Omega 3 fish oils because they can help protect against bone loss through the postmenopause.[9] These and the other recommendations will not only help prevent osteoporosis, but also heart disease and any other inflammation you may have present in your body, such as in your joints.

GET ENOUGH VITAMIN B

Research has also shown that high homocysteine levels (see page 205) are linked to an increased risk of osteoporosis and in one study women with high homocysteine levels had twice the risk of hip fractures compared to women with low levels,[10] so make sure you are getting enough of the B vitamins, which help to detoxify homocysteine (see chapter 14).

INCREASE YOUR INTAKE OF ANTIOXIDANTS

We know that certain nutrients are important in osteoporosis prevention including calcium, magnesium, boron and vitamin D but it is also thought that antioxidants are important for bone health.

One study proposed a theory of how oestrogen loss causes osteoporosis by concluding that a deficiency of the hormone lowers the antioxidants in osteoclasts (the cells that promote bone absorption), which increases their activity.[11]

Experts now believe that an increased intake of fruit and vegetables rich in antioxidants may improve bone health and reduce the risk of osteoporosis. One study showed that having good levels of certain antioxidants called carotenoids, found in fruit and vegetables, correlated with bone mineral density in postmenopausal women.[12] Experts also suggest that taking antioxidants in supplement form may reduce the risk of osteoporosis.

These findings clearly support the arguments for eating more fruit and vegetables (which also make the body more alkaline, a key factor in the prevention of osteoporosis) to lower the risk of osteoporosis.

One interesting piece of research focused on onion consumption in women aged 50 years and older. They showed that women who consumed onions once a day or more had a bone density that was 5 per cent greater than women who only consumed onions once a month or less. Their conclusion was that in older women who consume onions frequently they could decrease their risk of hip fracture by more than 20 per cent compared to women who never eat onions.[13] I don't know why they selected onions in particular but it is possible that those women eating onions were also more likely to be better vegetable eaters in general. So this isn't to say go and eat lots of onions; the important thing is to go for a good variety of all the vegetables, and fruit too.

VITAMIN K

It is well known that green leafy vegetables such as cabbage, cauliflower, kale and broccoli are healthy foods but did you know that these vegetables can also help keep bones strong? This is not only because some of them contain calcium, but also because they are good sources of vitamin K. Avocados and kiwis are also good sources of vitamin K.

Vitamin K is a fat-soluble vitamin that plays an important role in blood clotting. There are two kinds of vitamin K: K1 and K2. K1 is synthesised by plants and vegetables and K2 by gut bacteria and is also found in fermented cheeses and natto (fermented soya beans). Vitamin K is an integral part of bone mineralisation and is needed to make a protein that's essential for bone formation. It is important in the utilisation of calcium and recently has also been shown to be helpful for heart disease. Vitamin K can help to stop deposits of calcium in the walls of blood vessels.

One study found that those who consumed moderate or high amounts of vitamin K (nearly all from vegetables) had a 30 per cent lower risk of hip fractures than women consuming little or no vitamin K.[14] This held true even when other factors affecting bone health, such as calcium and vitamin D, were taken into account. It didn't take much vitamin K – about 100 to 150mg a day – to achieve this protective effect. As an example, one portion of kale (3½oz/100g) gives you 500mg of vitamin K.

Supplementing with vitamin K has also been shown to reduce fracture incidence in postmenopausal women.[15]

The K2 form of vitamin K is also thought to play an important role in heart health as it may help stop calcification in the arteries. K2 remains in the blood for longer than K1 and the body can use it much more easily so it is thought to be a better choice if taken as a supplement.

NOTE

Do not take vitamin K if you are on warfarin, a blood thinner, because vitamin K can interfere with its action.

TAKE A GOOD PROBIOTIC

If you have been diagnosed with osteopenia or osteoporosis I recommend that you take a good probiotic (see page 223) as it will not only help your body manufacture vitamin K in the digestive system but also these beneficial bacteria help your body absorb calcium. Even if you take calcium for your bone health it is only any good if you can absorb it and these friendly bacteria help to support this absorption. (Take a probiotic with at least 22 billion organisms per daily amount. The one I use in the clinic is called Advanced Probiotic Plus; see www.natural healthpractice.com) We know that probiotics not only improve calcium absorption but also increase bone mineral density.[16]

CALCIUM AND VITAMIN D

Calcium and vitamin D are important for your bone health as they reduce the risk of fractures[17] and have a positive effect on bone density,[18] so you need to keep taking these all the time (see page 222 for details of doses).

HRT AND SERMS

If you have been taking HRT, it is likely that you will be asked to come off it after five years. However you may be seeking a medical approach to be used alongside the nutritional recommendations to prevent osteoporosis. Due to the known risks of HRT, it is not recommended for the long-term prevention of osteoporosis. Instead, scientists have developed new drugs called SERMs, which are aimed at postmenopausal women.

SERMS (SELECTIVE OESTROGEN RECEPTOR MODULATORS)

As the name implies, these drugs selectively stimulate oestrogen receptors in parts of the body where that stimulation would be useful, for example, in the bones and brain, and block the stimulation in areas where it could be dangerous, such as the breast. There are two SERMs I'd like to discuss here.

The most well-known SERM is tamoxifen, which is used to treat and prevent breast cancer because it works as an anti-oestrogen to the breast cells. However, a side effect is that it worsens hot flushes and increases the risk of DVT (deep vein thrombosis), and can also stimulate the oestrogen receptors in the womb increasing the risk of womb cancer.

There is now a SERM called raloxifene, which is licensed to prevent spine fractures caused by osteoporosis. It has been shown to increase bone mineral density and to reduce spine fractures but does not reduce the risk of fractures in any other sites on the body such as the hip, ankle or wrist.[19]

It would therefore only be worthwhile using raloxifene if you knew from a bone density scan that you had low bone density or osteoporosis in the spine. If the bone density in your spine is good but you have a problem in your hip then there is no point in taking raloxifene because it will not help your particular situation and you need to think about other drugs that will target the hip (see below).

Also, as with any drug, you need to weigh up the risks versus the benefits of taking it.

The benefits are:

- it reduces the risk of breast cancer
- it prevents spine fractures
- it does not increase the risk of womb cancer like tamoxifen does.

The side effects associated with raloxifene are:

- increased hot flushes
- leg (calf) cramps
- DVT
- pulmonary embolism (blood clot that travels to the lung and can be fatal)
- headache/migraine
- nausea/vomiting
- thrombophlebitis (inflammation of a vein).

OSTEOPOROTIC DRUGS

Instead of the SERMs mentioned above you may have been prescribed a drug specifically for osteoporosis. The most commonly used ones are called bisphosphonates and they have a number of different brand names (common ones are Fosamax and Actonel). There are also now less expensive generic versions of the drugs, such as alendronic acid, which are meant to be chemical equivalents of the branded ones. Bisphosphonates can be taken by mouth once a week or some once a month. There are some that are given as an injection every three months or as an infusion (a drip) once a year. Bisphosphonates are proven to reduce the risk of fractures in postmenopausal women.[20]

HOW DO BISPHOSPHONATES WORK?

Bisphosphonates work by stopping the loss of old bone so bone density increases, but this is achieved by holding on to old bone rather than by increasing new bone. My concern is that this effect seems fine to begin with because bone density increases but after four to five years of taking this drug it never leaves the body. When bone becomes too dense, it can actually become more brittle, with research showing that women whose bone density had increased after taking a bisphosphonate for seven years had three times more fractures than during the first three years of taking it.[21]

Research highlighted the fact that although the bisphosphonates improve bone quantity, after four years of use they can affect the bone quality and have a negative effect by increasing the risk of fractures.[22]

So when should you stop taking them? The research shows that because the bisphosphonates accumulate in bone they can continue to be released for years and that when stopped after five years they will still give protection against fractures for another one to two years. A paper in the *Journal of Clinical Endocrinology and Metabolism* has suggested that 'patients at mild risk might stop treatment after five years and remain off as long as bone mineral density is stable and no fractures occur. Higher risk patients should be treated for ten years, have a holiday of no more than a year or two, and perhaps be on a non-bisphosphonate treatment during that time.'[23]

SIDE EFFECTS

Unfortunately there are side effects from taking the medication. Oral bisphosphonates have to be taken on an empty stomach at least 30 minutes before eating or drinking and you must stay upright the whole time. Even doing this, many women experience digestive side effects including inflammation of the oesophagus (food pipe) and sore throats. Some complain of aches and pains in joints and muscles and irregular heartbeats. You should be careful about starting on this kind of medication if you already have digestive problems such as indigestion.

With the injections and infusions, the most common side effects are flu-like symptoms such as muscle aches and high temperature, which usually subside in a few days after the treatment.

The other side effect, which has come to the attention of not only the women taking the bisphosphonates but also dentists, is the possibility of osteonecrosis of the jaw (commonly known as jaw rot). The concern is that if you are on bisphosphonates and need invasive dental treatment, such as dental implants or a tooth extraction, then the ability of the bone to heal could be compromised as the cells in the jaw are destroyed. It is thought that the problem is mainly connected to treatment of bisphosphonates given by tablet rather than injection. I would suggest, though, that if you are thinking of going on a bisphosphonate (oral or injection/infusion) that you have a thorough dental examination before you start the drug and have any invasive dental work done, if you can, ahead of time. The Medicines and Healthcare Products Regulatory Agency (MHRA) in the UK suggest that if you are on bisphosphonates and also have other problems such as poor oral hygiene, chemotherapy, steroid treatment or cancer you should avoid invasive dental work.

However, there is no point in stopping the bisphosphonates because you need invasive dental work as there is no research to show that it will reduce the risk of osteonecrosis of the jaw.

OVERPRESCRIBED?

Another important topic is the possible overprescribing of osteoporotic drugs. Research shows that the benefits of using drugs to treat osteopenia – low bone density – but calling it pre-osteoporosis have been very much overstated and exaggerated[24] and it is encouraging unnecessary treatment in millions of low risk women. I would suggest that if you have been diagnosed with osteopenia that you follow the dietary and supplement recommendations in this section, have the relevant tests (especially vitamin D) and then retest your bone density in a year's time to see what the difference is before you embark on drugs you would be on for life.

OTHER DRUGS FOR OSTEOPOROSIS

Other drugs used for osteoporosis are calcitonin (inhibits the cells that break down bone) and calcitriol (which helps the metabolism of calcium into the bones). Newer drugs include Protelos (strontium ranelate), which has a dual action in that it not only stops the breakdown of old bone but helps to build new bone. It is taken as a powder but unfortunately contains an artificial sweetener. It does reduce the risk of fractures[25] and does not cause the same digestive side effects as the bisphosphonates but can increase the risk of clots. Some women have also experienced a severe allergic reaction to this drug and the symptoms can include a skin rash, mouth ulcers, swollen glands or a fever. If you experience any of these symptoms the recommendation is to stop the drug immediately and then see your doctor.

The drug used for extreme cases of osteoporosis is Forsteo (teriparatide), which is expensive and is self-injected daily for 18 months. It works by encouraging bone to grow at a faster rate. It does reduce the risk of fractures and is normally taken with calcium and vitamin D.[26] Side effects can include nausea, headaches, dizziness and limb pains.

A new drug called Prolia (denosumab) is now available on the NHS. It is given as a six-monthly injection and works in a different way to bisphosphonates and the other osteoporotic drugs on the market. Prolia stimulates the immune system to block rank ligand, which is a protein that causes osteoclast activity, the cells that break down bone. Research has shown that Prolia can reduce the risk of a spinal fracture by 66 per cent and the risk of a hip fracture by 40 per cent.[27]

But as with any drug, there are trade-offs with the side effects, which can include back pain, high cholesterol and bladder infection. Severe reactions may include low blood calcium and skin reactions, as well as osteonecrosis of the jaw (see page 220).

SUPPLEMENTS FOR OSTEOPOROSIS AND OSTEOPENIA

If you have been diagnosed with osteopenia or osteoporosis, then you will need extra bone nutrients such as calcium and vitamin D on top of what is in your multi. Do not just focus on calcium and vitamin D because other nutrients like magnesium, zinc and boron are just as important for bone health. Take the following extra supplements:

Calcium (500mg calcium citrate): Calcium carbonate is one of the most difficult forms of calcium to absorb and if the calcium does not end up being deposited in your skeleton (where you want it to go), it can create calcification in your heart and breast.

Magnesium (900mg magnesium citrate): Magnesium is the second most abundant mineral in your bones after calcium so it is an important mineral for bone health. In fact, most women I see in the clinic are not deficient in calcium but they are in magnesium. Magnesium helps your body use calcium efficiently.

Vitamin D (300ius as vitamin D3 not D2): A vital nutrient for the absorption of calcium and helps to make sure that calcium ends up in your bones and is not deposited somewhere else in your body.

Zinc (15mg): Zinc works with vitamin D to help boost calcium absorption.

Boron (1mg): Improves the absorption of calcium by converting vitamin D to its active form.

(I use a good combination of all these nutrients in a supplement called Osteo Plus from the Natural Health Practice, www.naturalhealthpractice.com. See Useful Resources page 283.)

A good probiotic – containing at least 12 billion bifidobacteria strains and 10 billion lactobacillus acidophilus – will help with the efficient absorption of calcium and the manufacture of vitamin K2. Buy one that does not need refrigerating and if it has added prebiotics then that would be a bonus as the prebiotics are the 'food' for the probiotics (see NHP's Advanced Probiotic Plus at www.naturalhealthpractice.com).

If you would like to read more about osteoporosis, see my book *Osteoporosis – How to Prevent, Treat and Reverse It* (Kyle Cathie).

CHAPTER 16

OTHER HEALTH RISKS AFTER THE MENOPAUSE

Keeping yourself in the best of health with a good diet and supplements that are suited to the postmenopause is very important.

However, beyond the menopause there are certain health conditions that you should be aware of. The two biggest health risks past the menopause are heart disease and osteoporosis. Cardiovascular disease is the biggest killer, so you want to put the emphasis on keeping your heart healthy; and one in two women will get osteoporosis, so you need to keep your bones in good shape (see chapter 15).

In this chapter I will cover the main health issues that can affect women beyond the menopause and suggest specific nutrients that you can add to your maintenance programme for certain health problems. For conditions such as osteoporosis it is worth staying on the extra nutrients long term for your bone health but for other conditions such as joint pains, once your symptoms are gone, you can drop the extra nutrients and just stay on the maintenance programme outlined in chapter 14.

If you want individual help then do contact my clinic (details on page 283).

YOUR HEART

We tend to think of heart disease as being more of a problem for men but more than half of all women over 50 will die from heart disease. Statistics from the British Heart Foundation show that heart disease is the UK's biggest killer and is the leading cause of premature death, which is death before the age of 75.

Heart disease is a bigger killer for women than breast cancer (one in seven for heart disease compared to one in nine for breast cancer) but many more women fear breast cancer and will not necessarily think about heart disease as a woman's issue. In fact, you are twice as likely to die from heart disease as a woman than any form of cancer.

Cardiovascular or heart disease is an umbrella term to include coronary artery disease, angina, heart attack, stroke and high blood pressure. Although as women heart disease is our biggest killer, on a very positive note it is preventable.

Up until the menopause, oestrogen not only helps to protect your bones but also your heart. It is thought that oestrogen helps to maintain high levels of HDL (good cholesterol) and low levels of LDL (bad cholesterol) and that this 'female' hormone helps to keep your blood vessels healthy and blood flowing easily. Unfortunately, this means that in the postmenopause stage of your life, when oestrogen declines, there is a higher risk of heart disease.

It should be noted that a woman's symptoms for a heart attack can be very different to those of a man and can be easily missed or even dismissed as indigestion or heartburn. Women can feel just a mild, uncomfortable sensation in the chest with a dull or heavy feeling and the chest pain can feel like indigestion.

THE TRUTH ABOUT SATURATED FAT

It has become apparent over the years from working in the clinic, and doing the research for lectures and books, that in fact *saturated fat does not cause heart disease.* Nor does it make you overweight (see chapter 10). I know this contradicts all the messages you have heard over the years but the fact is that people are reducing their fat intake, buying low fat and reduced fat foods, and yet there is a worsening health crisis in the UK.

So what is going on? We have been focusing on the same wrong message and if that message does not change the health crisis will just get worse. Study after study has shown that reducing fat intake makes no difference to heart disease risk. In fact, a large study of over 48,000 women followed over 12 years showed that even when women reduced their total fat intake to 20 per cent of their total calorie intake, there was no reduced incidence of heart attack, stroke, bowel cancer, breast cancer or any form of heart disease.[1]

Research in 2010, which combined the results of 21 studies (a staggering 347,747 people followed for up to 23 years), stated 'there is no significant evidence for concluding that dietary saturated fat is associated with an increased risk of coronary heart disease, stroke and cardiovascular disease'.[2]

When it comes to weight loss, when researchers compare a low-fat to a low carbohydrate diet, the low carbohydrate diet comes out streets ahead – with the participants on the low carbohydrate having significantly more weight loss at six and twelve months, significantly higher HDL (good cholesterol) and lower triglycerides (fat in the blood).[3]

The message of 'saturated fat raises cholesterol' and 'cholesterol causes heart disease' therefore 'saturated fat causes heart disease' has become so ingrained that everyone still believes that 'fat makes you fat'. It has been accepted for so long that I suspect that it is not easy for healthcare professionals to admit that maybe this is not correct.

I believe that fat is not the culprit but *refined carbohydrates and the sugar produced from them.* If you think back to that roller-coaster of blood sugar swings I described on page 49, higher levels of insulin will make your liver produce more total cholesterol and more LDL (bad cholesterol). The high insulin will create free radicals, which will oxidise the fats that can form plaque in the arteries. The cortisol released when the blood sugar levels suddenly drop creates inflammation and you then end up with a recipe for disaster. And that inflammation then increases the risk of not only heart disease, but also osteoporosis, Alzheimer's, cancer, high blood pressure, stroke and diabetes.

HOW CAN YOU KNOW IF YOU ARE AT RISK OF HEART DISEASE?

There are a number of factors that can increase your risk of heart disease and these include a family history of heart disease or stroke, being overweight, too little exercise, high blood pressure (see page 234), stress and smoking.

The most obvious way to measure risk of heart disease is normally thought to be cholesterol and a common treatment for lowering cholesterol today, when linked to heart disease, is with the use of drugs called statins.

Is cholesterol really the cause?

Your body needs cholesterol, that's why it produces it. Your liver actually produces 80 per cent of the cholesterol in your body, only 20 per cent comes from your food. Cholesterol is present in all your cell membranes; your body uses it to make sex hormones (like oestrogen) and stress hormones (like cortisol) and also needs cholesterol for the manufacture of bile and vitamin D. Your brain needs cholesterol; it is crucial for it to function properly. Cholesterol has been given a bad name but it is essential for life.

As with anything in nature, it is always a question of balance; for example you don't want to have high blood sugar and you don't want to have low blood sugar. The same goes for cholesterol.

The interesting thing about cholesterol is that it can't travel around your body on its own. In order to get to your cells, it is carried in your blood by combining with a protein, called a lipoprotein (lipo stands for fat). It is the LDL (low density lipoprotein, often called 'bad' cholesterol) that carries the cholesterol to our cells and then it is removed and taken back to the liver by HDL (high density lipoprotein, 'good' cholesterol). If you have too much LDL and not enough HDL, then the cholesterol can be deposited on inflamed artery walls causing furring of the arteries (atherosclerosis), which can lead to blocked arteries. Note the word 'inflamed', which I will come back to shortly.

Research has shown that LDL is not a culprit on its own but becomes a problem when it is oxidised, so having enough good antioxidants from your diet and supplements is important at this stage in your life, as is being careful about too much iron. Women tend to think that if their energy is low they could be anaemic and should take iron. But iron is odd in that it can have both good and bad effects on your health. Iron is needed for energy as it makes red blood cells and haemoglobin and transports oxygen around your body. But stored iron (known as ferritin) produces free radicals that can destroy healthy cells and speed up ageing. You only lose iron when you bleed and before the menopause you will have lost iron each month during your period. However, at this stage in your life you are not having a menstrual cycle and therefore not losing any iron – you can even end up storing it. I advise you to get your haemoglobin and ferritin levels checked and only take iron supplements if you need them. If your iron levels are high, be careful about foods that are fortified with iron such as breakfast cereals.

I don't think cholesterol on its own causes heart disease and I have major concerns about using statins to lower cholesterol, especially in women (see below). One study looked at over 130,000 patients admitted to hospital with a heart attack and found they did not have high cholesterol but in fact had lower levels than normal.[4] This was also confirmed by another study looking at levels of LDL (bad cholesterol), showing that those patients with the lowest levels of LDL had twice the death rate three years later.[5]

Much research has shown that there is no difference in the heart disease rates in people with normal versus high cholesterol levels and that the highest levels of cholesterol are not linked with plaque in the arteries (atherosclerosis) and that people with the lowest levels of cholesterol can still have atherosclerosis.

What about statins?

Statins are cholesterol-lowering drugs that work by acting on the liver to reduce its production of cholesterol. With any drug you need to weigh up the risks versus the benefits. There are side effects with statins, which can include digestive upsets such as diarrhoea and flatulence, fatigue, nausea, liver problems, sleep disturbances and headaches. Statins can also cause memory loss, muscle pain, night cramps and sexual problems.

The memory loss and changes in brain function including intelligence, depression and even thoughts of suicide are emerging from the research as some of the more drastic side effects of statins. Your brain uses cholesterol to release neurotransmitters, chemicals in the brain, and people with very low levels of cholesterol (lower than 4mmol/l) are more likely to die from strokes, cancer, liver disease, lung disease and suicide.

Other research has shown that even though the statins lower cholesterol it does not change the death rate from heart disease but significantly increases the risk of cancer.[6]

Also, the French paradox is well known where they seem to eat a diet high in saturated fat and yet have low rates of heart disease. One study even compared the effectiveness of the Mediterranean diet to statins in preventing heart attacks and found that the diet was three times more effective than the drug.[7]

Statins and women

On top of my general concerns about statins and their side effects, research does not show that they are effective for women. Clinical trials on women taking statins who already have heart disease have not been shown to increase life expectancy at all and, in women with a lower risk, statins have not prevented heart attacks or strokes.[8] Unfortunately, women taking statins have shown an increased risk of breast cancer at the same level that would be expected from taking HRT.[9]

It should not be assumed that if a drug works on men it will have a similar effect on women. We also know that low dose aspirin makes no difference to the prevention of heart disease in women so if you have been told to take aspirin for this reason you need to think again as it will not help to prevent heart attacks but can cause internal bleeding.[10]

If you are taking statins then you should know that they not only reduce your liver's production of cholesterol but also reduce the production of co-enzyme Q10. Co-enzyme Q10 is contained in nearly every cell of your body. It is important for energy production in your cells and is vital for heart and muscle function. Not having enough co-enzyme Q10 makes you age faster and can accelerate DNA damage. Even just two weeks on a statin can cause a significant decrease in co-enzyme Q10 levels.[11] Co-enzyme Q10 can help to increase HDL (good cholesterol) and also lower blood pressure.[12]

CASE STUDY: ELAINE'S STORY

Elaine was 46, with a regular menstrual cycle, and with a family history of high cholesterol. Her mother, sister and father all had high levels but only her father was on medication. A normal level of cholesterol is 5 mmol/L and under so when Elaine's blood test by her GP showed her cholesterol to be at 7 mmol/L she was given statins. The month after taking the statin her periods stopped and she did not have another period for 18 months while still taking the statin. Her cholesterol measured during this time was down at 2.3. She then stopped taking the statin and, the next month, her periods returned to normal. Her cholesterol level is now 6.7 and she is being urged to take statins again. Remember that cholesterol is the starting block for the sex hormones so when her cholesterol was reduced to such a low level at 2.3, her body did not have enough to produce the hormones necessary for her to have a cycle. There are always consequences when we interfere with something in the body; it is just that we don't always see it in such an obvious way.

INFLAMMATION, THE REAL CULPRIT

Inflammation is the real cause of heart disease and has been dubbed the silent killer – it is linked to not only heart disease, but also cancer, Alzheimer's and diabetes.

It is interesting that findings suggest when statins do have a beneficial effect it is in an anti-inflammatory way, rather than by the lowering of cholesterol.[13]

Inflammation can be a life-saving mechanism. If you are cut or injured, the pain, heat, swelling and redness produced around the wound shows that your body is mobilising its immune defences to make your blood clot faster so you don't bleed to death, to be ready in case bacteria get into the wound, to release histamine to slow down foreign substances and to release substances called cytokines to create more inflammation to destroy pathogens (bacteria and viruses). It is as if your body is on fire.

The problem occurs when there is chronic inflammation going on in your body, day in, day out, caused largely by lifestyle factors, including stress, poor diet, lack of exercise, infections, toxins, smoking and too much alcohol. Added to this is the effect of the menopause, which makes women more prone to inflammation. As oestrogen production declines from the ovaries, and we go through the menopause and out the other side, there is a rise in substances (called cytokines), which can cause inflammation.[14]

When cholesterol is travelling around your arteries it only gets deposited in your blood vessels if your arteries are inflamed. The inflammation damages the lining of the blood vessels, making it easier for fatty deposits to stick. Over time this fatty deposit (or a clot) can come away from the blood vessel and can cause a heart attack if it blocks the blood supply to the heart, or a stroke if it blocks the blood supply to the brain.

An interesting study showed that daily treatment with a statin reduced the rate of heart problems and deaths in people whose cholesterol was healthy.[15] These people would not have been prescribed statins normally because they did not have high levels of cholesterol but what they did have were high levels of a protein called C reactive protein. (The effects of the statin were small, giving a 94.9 per cent chance of surviving the next five years compared to 94.3 per cent if they weren't taking the drug and in my view the risks of taking the statins, especially for women, outweigh the benefits.)

C reactive protein is a marker of inflammation and is tested by blood. So you could have normal levels of cholesterol but high levels of C reactive protein, in which case you could take action to work on lowering the inflammation with nutrition and lifestyle changes before your arteries start to fur up.

As well as C reactive protein, there is another substance that can be measured in blood, and high levels are linked to increased inflammation, free radical damage, damaging and thickening the artery walls and increasing the risk of blood clots. This is homocysteine, which is an amino acid, and high levels have been linked to heart disease, Alzheimer's and osteoporosis. Homocysteine is produced in the body as it breaks down an essential amino acid called methionine. The homocysteine should be successfully detoxified and excreted by the body but if this does not happen it can increase inflammation. The B vitamins (in particular, B6, B12 and folic acid) control this detoxification so if you have deficiencies you can end up with high levels of homocysteine. In one clinical trial, giving extra B vitamins not only reduced homocysteine levels but also improved insulin resistance and the health of the blood vessels.[16]

Having a good level of friendly gut bacteria is also important in controlling inflammation. We know that unfriendly gut bacteria cause inflammation so follow the diet and supplement recommendations on page 203 to make sure you are getting enough of the good bacteria.

Vitamin D (see page 236 for details of doses) also has a role to play in controlling inflammation. It can inhibit substances that cause inflammation and also help to boost those that are anti-inflammatory. It has also been shown to lower C reactive protein, which, as we have seen, is one of the markers of inflammation.[17]

The same is true for the Omega 3 fatty acids. As explained on page 27, these fatty acids have an anti-inflammatory effect on the body and are very important not only for general health but also in the prevention of heart disease. By increasing your intake of Omega 3 fatty acids you will decrease the substances that cause inflammation anywhere in the body.[18] In two clinical trials reported in the *Lancet*, fish oil (high in Omega 3) was found to be even better at reducing death or hospitalisation than statins.[19]

There are many other conditions that involve inflammation, such as arthritis and inflammatory bowel problems, and also where the immune system is on such alert that in the end it turns on itself and the inflammatory process attacks healthy cells, as in autoimmune disorders such as psoriasis, multiple sclerosis, lupus, rheumatoid arthritis and Crohn's disease.

I believe that inflammation is the cause and this manifests itself in different ways in different people, depending on their genetic make-up, lifestyle and nutrition.

HIGH BLOOD PRESSURE

Unfortunately, the possibility of having high blood pressure or hypertension becomes more likely with age as in the postmenopausal stage you do not have the protective effects of oestrogen. Before the age of 45 more men than women suffer from high blood pressure but from the age of 65, high blood pressure is more common in women than men.

Two numbers are used to measure blood pressure, for example 120 over 80. The first number relates to your systolic blood pressure, the pressure in your blood vessels when your heart beats. The second number is the diastolic pressure and relates to the pressure in your blood vessels when your heart rests. Both numbers are important. In general terms, these are the classifications for blood pressure:

120/80	Normal blood pressure
121/81–139/89	Mild hypertension (mild high blood pressure)
140/90 and over	High blood pressure (hypertension) that needs to be treated

See the chart opposite for the different readings:

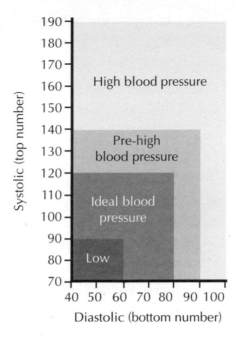

BLOOD PRESSURE CHART

This chart shows that both numbers do not have to be high for there to be a problem.

If the first number is over 140 you have high blood pressure no matter what the bottom number is and you need to take action.

If the second number is 90 or more then you have high pressure no matter what the top number is and you need to take action.

SYMPTOMS OF HIGH BLOOD PRESSURE

You may get symptoms such as headaches, blurred vision, nosebleeds, burst blood vessels in the eyes, tinnitus (ringing in the ears) or dizziness but alarmingly you may be one of the many sufferers who experience no symptoms at all.

It is estimated that as many as one in four women over the age of 50 may have high blood pressure and if it is not controlled it can put a strain on your heart and can cause kidney and eye damage, hardening of the arteries and increase your risk of heart attack and stroke. It is thought that three out of five cases of heart attacks in women are due to high blood pressure.

There are some easy to use and reasonably priced home blood pressure kits you can use to measure yourself. An arm blood pressure monitor is more accurate than a wrist one. If your reading is over 120/80 then take action immediately, see your doctor and put in place the dietary, lifestyle and supplement recommendations below. The sooner you do something about the problem the better, even if your blood pressure is only mildly elevated. Note that the following recommendations are also helpful for heart disease.

SUPPLEMENTS FOR HEART PROBLEMS, STROKE, HIGH BLOOD PRESSURE AND HIGH CHOLESTEROL

I have put these conditions together because often the same nutrients are helpful for each condition.

Omega 3 fish oils

It is important that you take Omega 3 fish oils in your maintenance programme (see page 204) because of their anti-inflammatory effect but they can also help to prevent blood clotting abnormally. The use of Omega 3 fish oils has been shown to reduce the risk of strokes[20] and to reduce the risk of coronary artery disease and heart attacks.[21]

Magnesium

Magnesium is also important for heart health and high blood pressure but you might find that you have enough (about 300mg magnesium citrate) in your multi (see page 205) and do not need to add in extra.

Vitamin D

It is so important that you are not deficient in vitamin D for your heart health.[22] You will have vitamin D in your multi but do get your level tested and if deficient add in an extra 400ius (as D3) and re-test three months later to make sure the level is back to normal. Also, if you have high cholesterol, make sure you have a blood test for vitamin D. Your body uses cholesterol to make vitamin D, so if your vitamin D level is low it can end up producing more cholesterol to manufacture more vitamin D. By correcting a vitamin D deficiency, you could reduce your cholesterol level.

(If you have difficulty getting a vitamin D blood test, contact my clinic, see Useful Resources page 283, and we can arrange for it to be done by post. We will then tell you what you need to take to correct it and when to re-test.)

Dose: 400ius as D3 per day.

Co-enzyme Q10

This vitamin-like substance, which reduces in your body as you get older, is important for keeping your heart healthy, lowering cholesterol and blood pressure.

Dose: 50mg per day.

HERBS

The same anti-inflammatory herbs recommended for arthritis (see page 256) can be helpful for heart health, but also include the following.

Garlic

There is a particular form of garlic that I recommend called Aged Garlic, which is a concentrated form of organic garlic. More than 350 scientific studies have been completed on Aged Garlic, focusing on heart disease, high blood pressure, lowering cholesterol, immune-boosting effect, brain function and its anti-cancer effect.

Dose: 1,000mg per day.

Hawthorn

The leaves, flowers and berries of the hawthorn are a general tonic for the cardiovascular system. Hawthorn is perhaps the best-known herbal medicine used in the treatment of mild high blood pressure. It improves heart function and helps treat congestive heart failure, irregular heartbeats and angina. It lowers blood pressure by relaxing and dilating artery walls. It is the ideal herb to use in the early stages of high blood pressure.

Dose: 300mg per day.

Dandelion

This familiar herb is a popular home remedy for fluid retention as it acts as a diuretic. By gently increasing urine flow dandelion helps to lower blood pressure.

Dose: 300mg per day.

DE-STRESS

Stress will cause inflammation and this can affect your heart and blood pressure. Try to find a method of relaxation that you enjoy whether it is meditation, yoga, walking, swimming or other exercise and do it daily or at least every other day. Getting a pet may help too. Research has shown that having a pet can protect against the effects of stress better than drugs designed to lower blood pressure.

BREAST HEALTH

The risk of breast cancer and other cancers increases the older we get but there is still a lot that can be done to work on prevention. This is important because, as we have seen (page 3), over 39 per cent of breast cancers could be prevented and only 5 per cent are due to a genetic predisposition.

The World Cancer Research Fund (WCRF) has focused on a number of factors that help to reduce the risk of cancer and even though this section is about breast health some of these factors will help to reduce our risk of other cancers so I will mention these too.

Recommendations from the WCRF include avoiding sugary drinks and limiting consumption of foods high in added sugar, low in fibre or high in salt, eating more of a variety of vegetables, fruits, wholegrains and pulses such as beans, and limiting consumption of red meats and avoiding processed meats. (This sounds like my hormone balancing diet which you will have read about in chapter 2.)

I discussed the importance of phytoestrogens in the diet on page 20 and these have also been picked out by the WCRF. As well as these factors, some of which I will expand on here, there are some others I would like to mention.

RECOMMENDATIONS FOR HEALTHY BREASTS
Maintain a healthy body weight
Stay as lean as possible without becoming underweight. This reduces the risk of all these cancers: breast, bowel, endometrial (womb), gall bladder, kidney, oesophagus and pancreas. Putting on 1½ stones (9.5kg) after menopause increases breast cancer risk by 18 per cent and women who shed 1½ stone (9.5kg) after the menopause cut breast cancer risk by more than 50 per cent[23] so follow the recommendations in chapter 10 for maintaining a healthy weight.

Reduce alcohol
Limit alcoholic drinks to no more than two a day for men and one for women. This reduces the risk of breast, bowel, liver, mouth and larynx and oesophagus cancers.

Exercise
Do at least 30 minutes each day. (See chapters 3 and 9 for ideas.) This reduces the risk of breast, bowel and endometrial (womb) cancers.

Get more vitamin D

I have already mentioned the benefits of vitamin D for anti-ageing and also how important it is in the prevention of osteoporosis. But research over the last few years has also shown how important having good levels of vitamin D is in relation to breast health.

Vitamin D promotes apoptosis, which is cell death or cell suicide. The process of apoptosis is very important because it is your body's way of eliminating unhealthy cells and without this process those old or unhealthy cells could continue to survive. Vitamin D has also been shown to stop the multiplication of malignant breast cells[24] and an article in the *American Journal of Public Health* has commented that vitamin D can halve the risk of developing cancer and that 'vitamin D supplementation could reduce cancer incidence and mortality at low cost'.[25] Make sure you follow the recommendations on page 80 about getting out in the sunshine and also if you have a strong family history risk or are worried about your breast health, it is worth having a vitamin D blood test. (If you need help to have this tested then do contact my clinic, see Useful Resources, page 283.)

Eat less red meat

One other aspect I would like to discuss in detail and which was picked up in the WCRF factors mentioned above is red meat. We know that eating more than one-and-a-half servings (4½oz/130g) of red meat a week can double the risk of breast cancer compared to three-quarters of a serving.[26] You could think this might be due to the saturated fat content of the red meat, but according to research the problem is certain carcinogenic chemicals that are formed when the meat is cooked. These are called heterocyclic amines (HCAs) and they increase the risk of both breast and bowel cancer. They are only found in cooked muscle meat (which includes not only meat but also chicken and fish, but would not be found in other animal proteins such as eggs) and the higher the temperature of the cooking the more of them are formed so frying, grilling and barbecuing produces the largest amounts of HCAs. Stewing, boiling and poaching are done at much lower temperatures and produce insignificant amounts of HCAs. I don't eat meat (of any kind) or poultry but eat fish (oily and white), cooked at lower temperatures.

Increase your fruit and vegetable intake

Increasing your fruit and vegetable intake is important generally but there is one group of vegetables that is really important for prevention of breast cancer. These are the cruciferous vegetables and include broccoli, Brussels sprouts, cabbage and cauliflower. They contain a substance called indole-3-carbinol, which helps your body eliminate excess oestrogen. (Not all breast cancers are dependent on oestrogen but many are so you want your body to detoxify oestrogen efficiently.) Just one-and-a-half cups of these vegetables a day (9oz/250g) can reduce your risk by 25 per cent.[27]

Include flaxseeds (linseeds) in your diet

Flaxseeds (linseeds) contain lignans, which help the successful detoxification of oestrogen through the digestive system.[28] Try to include one tablespoon of ground flaxseeds (linseeds) a day; this can be sprinkled on porridge, for instance.

BREAST CANCER AND DAIRY FOODS

There are two schools of thought on the impact of dairy foods on developing breast cancer or stopping a recurrence. One is that all dairy foods should be eliminated completely; the other is that eating dairy foods does not make any difference to the risk.

What does the evidence show? We know that there is nearly a four times difference in the incidence of breast cancer between Western women (133 per 100,000) and Asian women (39 per 100,000) and in the East the women eat very little (if any) dairy foods. They also eat more of other foods that in the West we do not eat as much of, such as phytoestrogens (see page 20), oily fish and seaweed.

Many studies have tried to answer this question about dairy and breast cancer and the results are not clear. Some research has said there is 'no evidence to support a significant link between intake of dairy products and breast cancer risk',[29] while other research suggests that meat is most associated with breast cancer risk, followed by milk and then cheese,[30] so the link may be animal fat rather than just dairy *per se*. The difficulty in getting a straight answer can also be due to the fact that it is not easy to isolate just one part of the diet and say whether there is a cause and effect. We all eat a variety of foods and we are also exposed to substances from the environment such as toxins and xenoestrogens (see page 103) and there are lifestyle issues to consider such as stress, exercise, smoking and alcohol.

My concern is that dairy products naturally contain a substance called IGF-1 (insulin-like growth factor) but the levels are high in milk from pregnant cows. As the name implies it is designed to stimulate growth and as humans we produce it in childhood to help us grow. Unfortunately IGF-1 is known to stimulate cells to divide and multiply and has been implicated in not only breast cancer, but also lung, colon and prostate cancer. IGF-1 also prevents cell death (apoptosis), which is a safety mechanism that causes a cell to die at the appropriate time allowing new cells to develop. If apoptosis is prevented then it could mean that abnormal cells are able to survive and flourish.

In the US, cows are given recombinant bovine growth hormone (rBGH), which not only increases milk production by up to 20 per cent but also increases the levels of IGF-1 by up to five times. rBGH is banned in the EU so it is not given to cows in the UK but dairy products imported from the US can contain it.

My other concern is that nowadays cows are milked while they are pregnant as milk is produced on a much larger commercial scale. During pregnancy, levels of hormones such as oestrogen are much higher so the dairy foods that we eat will contain high amounts of this hormone, which is a risk factor for breast cancer. Also, oestrogen levels will be even higher when the cow is milked during the later stages of pregnancy. I believe that it is not good to add even more oestrogen into our bodies along with the xenoestrogens we are exposed to from the environment (see page 103). It is estimated that milk from a cow in the late stages of pregnancy can contain up to 33 times more oestrogen than milk from a non-pregnant cow and as the study mentioned above stated in relation to the risk of ovarian and womb cancers, 'among dietary risk factors, we are most concerned with milk and dairy products, because the milk we drink today is produced from pregnant cows, in which estrogen and progesterone levels are markedly elevated'.[31]

You don't need to eat dairy foods to stay healthy and if you are worried about where you will get your calcium from, then see the list of calcium-rich non-dairy foods in the Appendix on page 279. Also, as already noted on page 211, when dairy is eaten as cheese it has an acidic effect on your body and will cause calcium to be leached from your bones, so this is not a good form of dairy after the menopause anyway. My suggestion would be that if you are going to eat dairy foods concentrate on taking them in the form of organic live natural yogurts. At least you will be getting some beneficial bacteria from the yogurt and it is one of the easiest forms of dairy to digest. As a substitute for milk, I use organic rice or soya milk on my breakfast cereal and use soya milk to make custard sweetened with maple syrup.

BREAST SCREENING

From the age of 50 until the age of 70 you will be invited every three years to have regular mammograms. A mammogram is an X-ray of the breasts and in order to get a clear picture each breast is compressed between two plates. A number of patients have said how painful the procedure is and some have had to repeat it a couple of times on the same day as the X-rays have not been clear enough.

I have had concerns about the benefits of mammograms since I wrote my first book *Natural Alternatives to HRT* in 1997 and my opinion has not changed; research that came out in 2010 has confirmed it. The difficulty I have always had is that we are employing a diagnostic tool that uses radiation, which in itself can trigger cancer. A study in 2006 confirmed this by showing that mammograms can actually trigger the disease in some women and can increase the risk by more than 50 per cent if the woman has a family history of breast cancer.[32]

An independent review of the NHS breast screening programme in 2010 (which has been running for 20 years)[33] has shown that more than 7,000 women a year are told they have breast cancer when they don't (false positives) and this then leads to unnecessary treatments such as biopsies and even surgery including mastectomies, not to mention all the anxiety and worry that is caused after being told you have cancer. Concerns were also raised in 2006 when it was shown that for every 2,000 women having mammograms, only one will have her life prolonged but ten would have unnecessary treatment.[34]

It has been calculated that if 1,000 women started having breast screening at the age of 50 and had a mammogram every three years only one would have her life saved through early detection and treatment of cancer by the time those 1,000 women would have stopped being screened at the age of 70. That might be okay to save one woman's life if there were no risks from the procedure but if the procedure itself could trigger cancer and the screening leads to women having breasts removed unnecessarily, then for me the benefits do not outweigh the risks.

This 2010 independent review says that the report by the Department of Health 'exaggerates the benefit, omits the harms and looks like propaganda aimed at persuasion'. The review concludes by saying 'there is no convincing evidence that it has saved lives. In fact, the effect of 20 years of screening in the UK is not visible in the mortality statistics. In contrast, there is solid evidence of serious and common harms, and the screening programme is very costly. Does this not mean that it is time for an impartial review of the justification for mammography screening?'

The other concern raised by this review is that many women are being treated unnecessarily for tumours that are in fact non-invasive or dormant and they would have gone to their graves dying of something else, never knowing they had a problem, had these tumours not been picked up by mammograms.

It does seem like a similar situation to the whole cholesterol, heart disease and saturated fat myth. When a concept or procedure is accepted by a large number of people, even though the concept or procedure may not be correct or beneficial, it is hard to change the status quo. Changing the common view means that some people have to admit they got it wrong.

How can you screen for breast cancer without using mammography?
Ultrasound breast scanning is an alternative to the mammogram and uses sound waves rather than X-rays to form a picture. It is the same scanning technique that is used in pregnancy. Sometimes women may have a mammogram and are then referred for a breast ultrasound scan because mammograms cannot detect all breast cancers and some abnormalities are not visible on a mammogram. Ultrasound is often used when women are on HRT as their breasts can still be quite dense from the use of oestrogen. In the UK, you would have to go privately for an ultrasound breast scan as you would only be referred for ultrasound on the NHS if it was needed after a mammogram.

The other possibility is infrared mammography (also called thermal mammography), which works on the scientific principle that for a tumour to grow it has to have a blood supply, so it creates blood vessels. Thermal imaging is used to detect changes in body temperature because the more blood vessels there are the more heat is generated. It can therefore show inflammation in the breast tissue and hormone dysfunction but it can't detect calcification or lumps so it has its limitations.

It is also useful for women to check their breasts at home, once a month; for many women it is their own self-examination that has picked up a worrying lump. It is best to do two examinations, one lying down and one standing up.

Lying down: Using a pillow, lie with your head and shoulders on the pillow. Lift your right arm and put it behind your head. Use your left hand to stroke the right breast and underarm and take note of any changes. Repeat on the other side.

Standing up: Looking at a mirror, lift both your arms above your head and check that both breasts look the same. Have a look at both nipples and check for any bumps or discharge and that the position of the nipples looks the same, namely that one isn't retracted (pulled inwards).

If you are unsure about changes that you see, then make an appointment to visit your doctor for an examination. Usually there is nothing to worry about but it is better to get any changes checked out than spend time being anxious about it.

SUPPLEMENTS FOR BREAST HEALTH

The maintenance programme on page 204 will give you a good combination of nutrients including antioxidants and Omega 3 fish oils. The Omega 3 fish oils are important because they are known to protect against breast cancer and can help to inhibit tumour growth[35] and the combination of the DHA in the Omega 3 oils plus carotenoids (like beta-carotene) in the multi can cut cancer risk in half.[36] Your multi should also contain good levels of folic acid as it is known that if you are taking in more than 345µg a day you have a 38 per cent lower risk of breast cancer than those women who have intakes of less than 195µg.[37]

Add these extra nutrients to your maintenance programme.

Vitamin D

Vitamin D should be included in your multi but if you have a family history or a personal history of breast cancer have a blood test to check your levels and add in extra vitamin D to correct a deficiency. (If you have difficulty getting a vitamin D blood test then get in touch with my clinic, see Useful Resources, page 283.)
Dose: 300ius of D3 per day.

Probiotics

These are important for your general health but they also help to control oestrogen by binding it in the gut and helping your body excrete it efficiently.
Dose: Aim for one containing 22 billion organisms. (A good one I use in the clinic is called Advanced Probiotic Plus, see www.naturalhealth-practice.com.)

VAGINAL DRYNESS, ITCHING AND URINARY TRACT INFECTIONS

These are problems that affect many women in the postmenopause and yet they find it difficult to talk about. Some women find intercourse so uncomfortable that it seems easier not to do it and this can have a devastating effect on relationships. Low levels of oestrogen cause changes in the vagina, making it drier and less elastic and the tissue can become much thinner and more inflamed so friction during intercourse can sometimes cause bleeding. For some women it feels like they have cystitis after intercourse because the entrance to the urethra can become bruised, causing inflammation.

Some women I have seen in the clinic have become so dry and sore that they can't even have a cervical smear because the nurse can't get the speculum into the vagina.

The pH of the vagina changes through the menopause. Before the menopause your vagina is usually acidic and this keeps infections at bay but the drop in oestrogen causes the vagina to become more alkaline, which means that you can be more prone to vaginal infections. Changes in the vaginal pH and the vaginal flora can predispose you to urinary tract infections, itching and vaginal infections.

If you are so sore and dry that intercourse becomes unbearable then it is better to use a medical approach first of all. There are topical oestrogens available, which are just used vaginally and come in the form of pessaries or cream. You would use this daily for about four weeks to plump up the tissue and then the aim would be to follow the supplement recommendations below to see whether the natural approach could take over.

There are different brands of vaginal oestrogen; the ones that contain oestradiol are the most carcinogenic so ask for the brands that just contain oestriol, a less potent form of oestrogen (for example Ovestin and Ortho-Gynest).

SUPPLEMENTS FOR VAGINAL DRYNESS, ITCHING AND URINARY TRACT INFECTIONS

Follow the maintenance programme on page 204 – the Omega 3 oils will be especially helpful as they control inflammation and also lubricate the body from the inside out.

The vitamin C mentioned in the maintenance programme is also crucial because it is important for the manufacture of collagen. You want to keep the walls of the vagina elastic in order to make intercourse more comfortable and reduce the amount of irritation and friction, which also reduces the risk of urinary tract infections. You also want to keep the urinary tract elastic and flexible, which can help to prevent stress incontinence and leakage. Having enough collagen is critical for this so make sure you take vitamin C every day.

Take these supplements on top of the maintenance programme:

Probiotic

Because of the change in pH of the vagina you want to make sure that you have good levels of beneficial bacteria in the digestive system, which can help to protect you against thrush, vaginal and urinary infections. Aim for one containing 22 billion organisms. (I recommend Advanced Probiotic Plus; see www.naturalhealthpractice.com.)

Natural lubricant

You can either use this instead of a vaginal oestrogen or use it when you have stopped using the vaginal oestrogen and you are finding intercourse more comfortable. Most of the lubricants on the market contain chemicals such as parabens that I would not want to recommend inserting into the vagina. The one I use in the clinic is appropriately called 'Yes' and is an organic lubricant that contains no preservatives or chemicals and is made from cocoa and shea butter. (It is available from www.naturalhealthpractice.com.)

Cranberries

If you are suffering from recurrent cystitis then cranberries can be extremely beneficial because they stop bacteria from attaching to the walls of the urinary tract. Using cranberry juice that is sweetened with sugar is not going to be helpful so you should either use an unsweetened cranberry juice (with no artificial sweeteners either) or, better still, take it in a concentrated dried form as a supplement.

Take a high dose of cranberry (3.6g) when you are having an attack and use a maintenance dose of up to 300mg to prevent the cystitis recurring.

LACK OF SEX DRIVE/LOW LIBIDO

Your sex drive may be low because intercourse is painful due to vaginal dryness and many women I see in the clinic have almost developed a phobia to sex, tensing up every time they have intercourse because it hurts so much. The first step is to follow the recommendations above to improve conditions in the vagina and make intercourse more comfortable again.

But you may have lost interest in sex completely. Indeed, many women tell me that they would rather read a book than have intercourse, but feel they ought to do something about it for the sake of their relationship.

There are many factors that can cause a drop in sex drive, including tiredness, stress, too much alcohol, depression and also low thyroid function, so see if you need to take action to make changes in any of these areas. Also think about your relationship; is it fundamentally good and is it just that your sex drive seems to have diminished or do you feel that there are underlying issues that need to be resolved?

The menopause is often termed 'the change' and many women I see in the clinic tell me they have only stayed in a relationship for the sake of the children and the time that the children leave home often coincides with the first years past the menopause. This stage is often a time for re-evaluation and many women will often pursue a new career or hobby because they have more time and some will make decisions about their relationships too. As one patient said to me, 'this HRT is wonderful; it is not Hormone Replacement Therapy but Husband Replacement Therapy!' It is worth considering counselling in order to talk through your feelings and help your partner understand what you are going through. Your partner may also be questioning life and future plans so you could decide to go for help alone or even together to talk openly about relationship concerns.

You may not feel so sexy and attractive because your body has changed and you have put on some extra weight since the menopause. Do follow the recommendations in chapter 10 if you are not happy about this extra weight, but remember that for most partners this is not an issue and will often be something that you think about and they don't.

One other important issue for a good sex life is your general health. Research has looked at how sexually active people are in mid life and older and it seems that many men *and* women who have good or excellent health are more likely to be sexually active compared to those of the same age in poor or only fair health. Those in good or excellent health were nearly twice as likely to report an interest in sex as those in poorer health, so it pays to look after yourself not only for your general health but your sexual health.[38]

Don't rule out a physiological reason for why you have low libido. It could be due to low thyroid function, as mentioned above, but it can also be caused by the change in hormones since the menopause. Oestrogen production is low after the menopause but testosterone can also be reduced. Women who have had their ovaries removed will often feel their sex drive has diminished because it is in the ovaries that testosterone is made. Testosterone is thought of as a 'male' hormone but women do produce it, though in much smaller amounts than men, which for some women reduces at the menopause to a low enough level to affect sex drive and reduce motivation and the feeling of 'get up and go'.

On the other hand, the sex drive of some women actually increases after the menopause. There can be a number of reasons for this: one is the freedom from the risk of getting pregnant and the need for contraception; another may be the start of a new relationship around this time; but in others it can be that as oestrogen levels decrease the testosterone they produce becomes more dominant. They are not necessarily producing more testosterone but the balance has shifted so in relation to the lowered oestrogen it seems like more.

You also produce androgens (male hormones) from the adrenal glands so if you are stressed or not eating well (on a blood sugar roller-coaster, which produces the stress hormones), then you may not be producing enough androgens and this decreases the sex drive.

SUPPLEMENTS FOR LACK OF SEX DRIVE/LOW LIBIDO

Make sure that you taking the maintenance programme of a good multi, Omega 3 fish oils and vitamin C. The multi will give you good levels of zinc, selenium and the B vitamins, which are important for sex drive. Zinc is crucial for the production of your sex hormones (which is why oysters have such a reputation as an aphrodisiac as they contain high amounts of zinc).

The multi will also contain vitamin E, which can help with vaginal dryness. The fish oils are important as they help to keep your body lubricated and soft, including the vagina. This is not a time to be on a low-fat diet. Vitamin C is crucial for the manufacture of collagen, which can help to keep elasticity and stretch in the vagina.

Take these supplements on top of the maintenance programme:

St John's wort (Hypericum perforatum)

This herb is known for its help with mild to moderate depression and for some women it can help with sex drive, especially if it is connected to feeling low.

Dose: 300mg two to three times a day.

Damiana (Turner aphrodisiaca)

This Central American herb can be useful for improving libido. You can tell even by the scientific name of the plant that it can act as an aphrodisiac.

Dose: 300–600mg twice daily.

Ginkgo biloba **(Ginkgo biloba)**

Ginkgo biloba can be useful in improving sex drive by improving blood flow to the sex organs and making them more sensitive.

Dose: 300mg per day.

EYES

At this stage in your life you need to pay particular attention to your eyes because age-related macular degeneration (AMD) is the leading cause of blindness for people over the age of 55 and women are more likely to develop AMD than men. AMD is a disease of the retina and causes loss of central vision, leaving only peripheral vision. The macula is a small area at the centre of the retina which allows you to see in front of you and to see colours. If the macula gets damaged, the central vision can be blurred, which makes reading and writing difficult.

TYPES OF AMD

There are two types of AMD – wet and dry. This is what the eye specialist (ophthalmologist) sees as they look at the macula; it does not describe how the eye feels.

Wet

New blood vessels grow abnormally beneath the macular and the blood vessels cause the macula to be scarred, preventing vision. Wet AMD makes up about 10 per cent of all AMD cases.

Dry

This is the most common type of AMD and develops very slowly over time with the normal tissue in the macula disappearing.

WHAT'S THE CAUSE?

Smoking, high cholesterol, obesity and poor diet have all been suggested as causes, and the one thing they have in common is that they cause inflammation and can create free radical damage, which will destroy cells anywhere in the body, including the eye. The Omega 3 fatty acids are concentrated in the retina (particularly DHA) and research has shown that higher levels of Omega 3 fish oil intake can reduce the risk of both wet and dry AMD by up to 35 per cent.[39]

SUPPLEMENTS FOR EYE HEALTH

For the health of your eyes you should focus on good levels of antioxidants, which you have in your multivitamin and mineral in the maintenance programme, plus the extra vitamin C (and get one which contains bilberry too), and the anti-inflammatory effect of the Omega 3 fish oils, which have been shown to reduce age-related macular degeneration. Nutritional supplements (antioxidants and zinc) given over a five-year period show a 25 per cent beneficial effect in reducing the risk of progression to advanced AMD in people with intermediate AMD.[40]

If you have a strong family history of AMD or are starting to experience problems, add in these extra supplements:

Lutein

Lutein is a carotenoid antioxidant that is concentrated in the retina and lens of the eye. Research has shown that giving 10mg lutein per day combined with a multivitamin and mineral supplement in a placebo-controlled trial resulted in significant improvements in visual function in people with AMD.[41]

Dose: 10mg per day.

Ginkgo biloba (**Ginkgo biloba***)*

This herb contains a number of antioxidants, for example ginkgo-flavonglycosides, which are helpful for eye health. Ginkgo also reduces abnormal blood clotting and improves blood flow.[42]

Dose: 100–300mg per day.

ARTHRITIS/JOINT PAINS

For some women joint pains and arthritis are their major symptoms as they go through the menopause and out the other side (it is sometimes termed 'menopausal arthritis') and this is due to the drop in oestrogen combined with getting older. But arthritis and joint pains are not inevitable, and even if your joints have started to be a problem, there is a lot you can do to improve the situation.

SUPPLEMENTS FOR ARTHRITIS/JOINT PAINS

The following programme of nutrients and herbs will work for any inflammation going on in the body that may cause arthritis and joint pains. It is also important that you pay particular attention to your diet, and eliminate foods and drinks that are causing your body to produce inflammation (see page 27). These extra nutrients are added in on top of the maintenance programme, which already includes good levels of the Omega 3 fish oils that are your most important anti-inflammatory supplement.

Glucosamine

Glucosamine is an amino sugar that forms an important part of the connective tissue within joints. It can help to rebuild cartilage. Research has shown that taking both glucosamine and Omega 3 fish oil is better than taking just glucosamine. As researchers have put it, 'in a randomised, controlled clinical trial with 177 patients with osteoarthritis, we could prove that the combination of glucosamine sulphate and Omega 3 fatty acids is superior to glucosamine alone'. In fact taking both supplements produced an 80 per cent reduction in pain score.[43]

Dose: 1,000–1,500mg per day.

Methyl suphonyl methane (MSM)

MSM occurs naturally in foods containing sulphur. It helps to maintain healthy connective tissue, keeping the joints flexible and reducing pain.

Dose: 3,000mg per day.

NOTE

You can get supplements where the glucosamine and MSM are combined together, which is more convenient than taking separate supplements. I recommend MSM combined with the glucosamine rather than chondroitin, another supplement that is said to help, as the research on chondroitin is not so convincing.

Vitamin D

Vitamin D is known to control inflammation and you will have some vitamin D in your multivitamin and mineral, but if you have severe joint and even muscle pains then I would suggest that you have a blood test for vitamin D levels (see page 283) and supplement with extra if needed. Research has shown that once you correct the deficiency the pain goes away.[44]

Dose: 300ius as D3 per day.

Herbs

A number of herbs can help ease arthritis and joint pains. A good anti-inflammatory combination would include turmeric, ginger, bromelain and white willow, taken in a herbal combination.

Aromatherapy

For osteoarthritis you could try a warming aromatherapy blend to ease muscle spasm, stiffness and poor circulation. Try blending three drops of ginger, three of lavender and four drops of black pepper in 20ml of carrier oil. For rheumatoid arthritis go for gentle, soothing anti-inflammatory oils: blend two drops of rose otto, two of yarrow and six drops of palmarosa oils in 20ml of carrier oil. Do not massage on the joints if there is pain; apply gently to the surrounding tissues instead.

WEIGHT MANAGEMENT

If you are gaining or losing weight quickly then you should always see your doctor to rule out any medical problem.

WEIGHT GAIN

You may find that you are gaining more weight at this stage in your life and also that the weight is sitting more around the middle. Unfortunately, your metabolism can slow down as you get older and this makes it easier for you to gain weight. Follow the recommendations in chapter 10 on how to lose weight without dieting and pay particular attention to getting your blood sugar levels even. If you are on the roller-coaster of blood sugar fluctuations and maybe missing meals or going long gaps without eating, this will slow your metabolism down further. Make sure that you are eating little and often.

You also need to be careful about eating too much since the older we get the less we really need to eat. Make sure that you are chewing well as this will improve digestion and absorption, but also because it takes your brain time to register that you are full. By slowing down as you eat you will end up eating less because your body will tell you when you have had enough.

Eating little and often will improve your metabolism, which means that you burn more fat instead of storing it. Also make sure that you include weight training as well as aerobics in your exercise routines; follow the suggestions on page 143. The more muscle you have on your body, the more fat you burn. It is a much faster way to lose weight and to maintain a good body shape than by aerobic exercise alone (such as walking or swimming).

It is important to manage your weight because being heavier than you should be can increase the risks of Type 2 diabetes, heart disease, cancer and high blood pressure, all degenerative diseases that we associate with getting older but which are not inevitable.

WEIGHT LOSS

There are some women I see in the clinic that no matter what they eat they don't gain weight. Some of these women are a healthy weight but others are not and they are too thin. It is important at any age not to be underweight but crucial after the menopause because of the risk of osteoporosis.

If you can't gain weight or are losing weight, read the section on being underweight on page 170. If it is a problem with digestion and absorption this is important to rectify because the food you eat is only as good as what you absorb, especially now you need to make sure that valuable minerals get into your bones and that your body is able to efficiently utilise the other nutrients from your food to keep your body healthy.

ALZHEIMER'S DISEASE AND DEMENTIA

Your brain is amazing. You are born with all the brain cells you will ever have – about 100 billion. Most of the brain does not regenerate as you get older except the hippocampus – an area for learning, which is important for long-term memory and spatial navigation, so you want to keep your brain as healthy as possible.

But brain function can change as we get older. The symptoms that are associated with a gradual decline in brain function such as loss of memory and difficulty in concentrating are described as dementia. The two main forms of dementia are Alzheimer's (the most common) and vascular dementia. Alzheimer's is caused by plaque and tangles developing in the brain. Plaque is formed by clumpy spheres that float between the neurons and prevent the transmission of messages to each other and the tangles actually choke the neurons from inside. Vascular dementia is a problem with the supply of blood to the brain.

The risk of dementia increases with age and affects about 5 per cent of people over the age of 65 but unfortunately is much more common in women.[45] I am going to concentrate on Alzheimer's in this section because it is the most common form of dementia. Not only does the risk of developing Alzheimer's increase with age but you can also have a higher risk if there is a family history of the disease. However, I suggest that no matter how old you are or your family history risk you follow the dietary and supplement recommendations below to reduce the possibility of developing the disease.

INFLAMMATION

As inflammation is now thought to be the cause of many degenerative diseases it is important to think about controlling inflammation in the brain in relation to reducing the risk of Alzheimer's disease. Make sure you are eating well and follow the hormone balancing diet on page 18 as this will help to reduce inflammation. Pay particular attention to keeping your blood sugar in balance because if you are on the roller-coaster of blood sugar swings, the increase in cortisol as your blood sugar drops can produce more inflammation. Also the uncontrolled glucose and insulin from that roller-coaster is going to produce AGEs (Advanced Glycation End Products, see page 76), which are toxic to your brain and will make it age faster and damage cells.

ALCOHOL

Watch your alcohol intake as it acts as a diuretic and will cause you to flush out valuable nutrients that your brain needs to function. Alcohol can stop your body converting the good fats into beneficial anti-inflammatory substances, which can cause more inflammation in the brain.

OMEGA 3 AND OMEGA 6

Make sure you are eating oily fish or taking flaxseed oil (linseed oil) if you are vegetarian as these are absolutely crucial for controlling inflammation. By increasing your intake of fish research indicates you may be able to reduce the risk of dementia by 60 per cent.[46]

There has been a great deal of research on the association between increased Omega 3 intake and a reduced risk of developing dementia including Alzheimer's disease, so Omega 3 fatty acids are important to include in your diet. Just as important is what to exclude or reduce from your diet. It has also been shown that too high amounts of Omega 6 fats coming from vegetable oils can increase the risk of dementia[47] and meat is also associated with an increased risk.[48]

Not only may the Omega 3 fatty acids reduce the risk of developing Alzheimer's disease but research has also looked at using it as a treatment. A double blind placebo-controlled trial showed that Omega 3 fatty acids were helpful for those people who already had mild Alzheimer's disease.[49] Those who had higher levels of blood EPA (eicosapentaenoic acid, found in oily fish, see page 30) tended to have better results on cognitive function.

Your brain is 70 per cent fat but it needs to have the right type of fat. Brain cells need to be flexible to function properly and your brain incorporates the fats you eat into the cell membranes; this is why the Omega 3 fats are so important. It is also important to eliminate the trans fats (see page 37) because the same negative effect they have on your heart also happens in your brain. These are hard fats, like a plastic; they make cells rigid so they lose their elasticity and flexibility.

Given how important it is to have good levels of Omega 3 fatty acids and to make sure that you are not having too much Omega 6 coming in from the diet, it would be helpful to have a blood test to check what your levels actually are (see Useful Resources page 283 for help in organising this). This would be especially important if you have a high family history risk of Alzheimer's.

DIETARY PATTERNS

Research has also focused on whether different dietary patterns can protect you and reduce your risk of developing Alzheimer's. A recent study of over 2,000 people over the age of 65 (without dementia) followed for four years, has shown that those who have higher intakes of salad dressing, nuts, fish, tomatoes, poultry, cruciferous vegetables, fruits and dark green leafy vegetables and lower intakes of dairy products, red meat, organ meat and butter have a strongly associated lower risk of Alzheimer's.[50]

ANTIOXIDANTS

Having good levels of antioxidants is also important in reducing the risk of Alzheimer's disease. Research has shown a 30 per cent drop in dementia risk among regular fruit and vegetable eaters[51] so the recommendation is to 'eat a rainbow' of fruit and vegetables, as each colour will give you different antioxidants.

Research has also looked at the use of antioxidant supplements in reducing the risk of Alzheimer's. One study showed that a combination of vitamin E (400ius) and vitamin C (500mg) helped to reduce the risk[52] and it is also known that taking antioxidant supplements can reduce the deterioration rate of Alzheimer's in people who have already been diagnosed.[53]

ACETYLCHOLINE

People with Alzheimer's have been found to have a shortage of the neurotransmitter acetylcholine in the brain and drugs that mimic acetylcholine are often used as a treatment. Acetylcholine is critical for memory and brain function.

Choline is a precursor (starting block) for acetylcholine and is contained in high amounts in egg yolks and is also found in soya and nuts, so these are good foods for boosting memory and brain function.

Lecithin, which is sold as a food supplement, is a source of choline and researchers have looked to see whether adding lecithin into the diet would help with slowing down the symptoms of dementia and Alzheimer's. Unfortunately, the evidence is not strong although the researchers say that 'a moderate effect cannot be ruled out'.[54]

HOMOCYSTEINE

All the risks associated with heart disease are applicable to Alzheimer's so it is important to also think of homocysteine, a toxic amino acid, when aiming to reduce the risk of Alzheimer's disease. We know that people with high homocysteine levels in the blood (over 14µmol/l) have double the risk of developing Alzheimer's.[55] Testing for homocysteine levels is done by a blood test and if you know that your levels of homocysteine are high you can take extra folic acid, B6 and B12, to reduce it and then re-test it in three months' time to make sure it has reduced to a healthy level, and then aim to maintain it.

LOOK AFTER YOUR TEETH

It is known that oral health is linked to heart health as research has shown that those with gum disease are more likely to have narrowing of the arteries. It is thought that the same mechanism could be happening in the brain. The thinking is that bugs that cause gum disease enter the bloodstream setting up an immune system reaction, which then produces inflammation and narrows the blood vessels in the heart and the brain. Research has shown that people with poor oral hygiene and bleeding gums are more likely to suffer with memory problems.[56] Make sure you have regular check-ups not only with the dentist but also the hygienist and get into a regular habit of flossing as well as brushing.

STOP SMOKING

Anything that is going to effect blood flow can have a detrimental effect on the brain, so it is never too late to stop smoking.

CONTROL STRESS

Ongoing stress is bad for your brain health. Stress causes the overproduction of cortisol, which increases the inflammatory response in your body. This will have a negative effect on the cells in your brain.

EXERCISE FOR YOUR MIND AND BODY

As well as eating well, make sure that you are physically active. It is good for your heart and to help prevent osteoporosis but it is also excellent for reducing your risk of Alzheimer's disease. Research has shown that being active in mid life at least twice a week can reduce or delay the onset of Alzheimer's even in those people with a strong family history risk.[57]

As well as being physically active keep yourself mentally active because it is known that people who are intellectually active can keep their mental function good right through their life.[58] Keep doing the crosswords and the Sudoku and even try learning a new language or a musical instrument. Think of your brain as a muscle; it is use it or lose it; so you want to keep your brain in training.

SUPPLEMENTS FOR ALZHEIMER'S DISEASE AND DEMENTIA

Make sure you are taking the maintenance programme of a good multivitamin and mineral (which will give you good levels of the B vitamins including folic acid and also antioxidants such as vitamin A and E), Omega 3 fish oils and vitamin C.

If you have an increased risk because of your family history or you have been told that you have mild Alzheimer's disease then add in the following on top of the maintenance programme:

Acetyl L-carnitine

This amino acid can help with the production of acetylcholine. Acetyl L-carnitine is able to cross the blood–brain barrier and get to the blood circulation in the brain. Research in mice has shown that a combination of nutrients including acetyl L-carnitine, alpha-lipoic acid and DHA (from fish oil) may be helpful in delaying the cognitive decline as we get older.[59]

Dose: 250–500mg per day.

Ginkgo biloba (Ginkgo biloba)

This herb is known for its ability to improve blood flow and circulation. So it has been suggested that it might be helpful in preventing or reducing Alzheimer's by maintaining good flow to the brain. Ginkgo also contains potent antioxidants that can control free radicals, which can damage cell membranes anywhere in the body including the brain. It is also suggested that ginkgo may help to protect nerve cells that are damaged in Alzheimer's.

Previous research on this herb has shown mixed results, but research in 2010 that looked at its effects not only on Alzheimer's but also on dementia in general, including vascular dementia, showed significantly better results compared to placebo in tests on cognition.[60]

Dose: 300mg per day.

INCONTINENCE

Incontinence is uncontrolled leakage or loss of urine and there are two main types of incontinence – urge and stress incontinence.

URGE INCONTINENCE

Urge incontinence, medically known as *detrusor dyssnergia*, is where there is a sudden need to pass urine and the woman may not be able to get to the toilet in time. It is usually caused by an overactive or irritable bladder. The bladder will often register the need to urinate when there is not much urine in there; it has become too sensitive and is telling that woman she needs to urinate when in fact she doesn't. The solution for urge incontinence is retraining the bladder to go longer between toilet visits and using distraction techniques so that more urine is passed at each visit. Begin by allowing yourself one trip to the toilet every hour for a week and then the following week extend the time between trips by half-an-hour. Continue until you can hold your urine for three hours at a time. This exercise teaches your bladder to hold more urine and become less sensitive when full.

Don't be tempted to drink less if you are prone to urge incontinence. Restricting your fluid intake will not stop the problem. In fact it can make things worse by producing highly concentrated urine that irritates the bladder. Drink lots of water instead. You'll know when you are hydrated if your urine appears clear to pale yellow. If it's dark yellow you aren't drinking enough.

Sometimes drugs are used in conjunction with the retraining to block the nerves in the bladder so it does not send out inappropriate messages to go to the toilet.

STRESS INCONTINENCE

Stress incontinence is the most common form of incontinence and causes women to leak urine when they laugh, cough, exercise or sneeze. It affects us more as women than it does men largely because of our anatomy and the menopause. The drop in oestrogen after the menopause causes the bladder muscles to lose their strength and flexibility. We also have a short urethra (the tube that runs from the bladder to the outside) at only 2in (5cm) in women compared to 7in (18cm) in men. Also the pressures during a vaginal birth can often weaken or stretch the tissues supporting the bladder making us more susceptible to problems after the menopause.

The first thing to do to try and improve stress incontinence is to perform pelvic floor exercises to help strengthen the pelvic floor.

Pelvic floor exercises (Kegels)

Kegel exercises can help combat incontinence. To find out which muscles you need to use, the next time you go to the toilet stop urinating in midstream by contracting your muscles; these are your pelvic floor muscles. Use these muscles to perform a Kegel, contract them and hold for a count of five and then relax. Repeat this ten times and do at least five times a day.

Devices to use alongside pelvic floor exercises

You can use certain devices to help maximise the benefit you get from the pelvic floor exercises.

One of these is a pelvic toner which is inserted into the vagina and helps you identify and isolate the correct muscles. You then exercise by squeezing against resistance.

The toner provides instant feedback to show you are squeezing correctly and, as you improve, you can increase the resistance in stages to make your exercise more demanding.

A pelvic toner does require effort from you so if you are looking for an easier approach choose an electric device.

One electric model (wireless) uses a mild electric stimulation that invigorates the pelvic floor muscles with no effort on your part.

(Both of these devices are available from www.naturalhealthprac-tice.com. For more information see the website.)

Surgery

Surgery is usually offered when the pelvic floor exercise and/or devices have not helped. The main aim of surgery is to support or tighten the muscles and other structures around the bladder.

The simplest form of surgery is the bladder neck injection, which only takes a few minutes under local anaesthetic. A natural (collagen, silicone or fat) or synthetic (Teflon) substance is injected around the neck of the bladder to help keep it closed. It has a success rate of about 70 per cent but may need to be repeated a few years later as the material may be broken up or absorbed by the body.

Another method is the use of tension-free vaginal tapes, where a synthetic sling is inserted, under local anaesthetic, to support the urethra and vagina. This technique has about an 80 per cent success rate.

Colposuspension is the most effective of the surgical procedures, with up to a 90 per cent success rate, but it is performed under general anaesthetic and is classed as a major operation. A cradle of stitches is made like a hammock to lift the bladder neck back into the correct position.

DIETARY RECOMMENDATIONS

The main emphasis with your diet is to eat as healthily as possible and make sure that you are eating enough foods that contain vitamin C and bioflavonoids (also called flavonoids). They help to preserve collagen and stop its destruction. Collagen is important for elasticity not only in skin but also in the tissues that support the bladder and vagina. Bioflavonoids are water-soluble plant pigments and they are found in a wide range of foods. So the recommendation is again to 'eat a rainbow'; the more different coloured fruits and vegetables you can eat will not only give you good amounts of vitamin C but also different kinds of bioflavonoids that will help with the manufacture of collagen.

It is important to make sure you drink enough liquid either in the form of straight water or herbal teas. But do not go overboard as of course the more you drink the more you will have to urinate out. Also be careful about too many drinks that actually act like a diuretic and cause you to pass more urine than you would normally – these can include caffeinated drinks and also alcohol.

SUPPLEMENTS FOR INCONTINENCE

Take the maintenance programme of a good multi, Omega 3 and vitamin C. The vitamin C is even more important in this situation for the manufacture of collagen; always go for the gentler ascorbate form of vitamin C (it will say magnesium ascorbate on the container) rather than ascorbic acid. Take 500mg twice a day.

Herbs can be really useful for helping with stress incontinence. The main herbs to use are horsetail (*Equisetum arvense*), which contains good amounts of silica that helps strengthen connective tissue generally in the body and also around the bladder. Silica is found in foods such as carrots, apples, onions, pumpkin, fish, almonds and unrefined grains.

Ladies' mantle (*Alchemilla vulgaris*) is also another useful herb for helping to strengthen connective tissue. Take 300mg twice a day of each of horsetail and ladies' mantle.

HAIR LOSS

This can be very distressing for women as it is such an obvious problem and it can shake a woman's self-confidence and cause depression and anxiety. It is normal to lose about 100 hairs a day as part of the cycle of hair growth. Hair is comprised of keratin, which is the same protein that is found in your nails.

It is important to rule out possible causes of hair loss so get your thyroid function checked and also iron levels (ferritin, your iron stores), as problems with either of these can cause hair to thin and fall out.

Also your hair, as with your nails, can be a reflection of your general health so make sure that you are eating well, drinking enough fluids and either eating enough oily fish or taking a fish oil supplement (see below), especially if your hair is dry, which can make it break easily. Include enough animal protein (like fish or eggs) and/or vegetable protein (such as nuts, seeds and beans) in your diet as hair is made up of a large percentage of protein. Being deficient in certain nutrients can also be a cause of hair loss so follow the supplement recommendations below.

Stress can also be a major factor in hair loss so have a look at what you can control in your life and take some extra supplements (see below) to lessen the toll on your hair and general health if you are under a lot of stress.

However, the change in hormones through the menopause may be what is causing your hair to thin on the top and at the sides. It is called androgenetic alopecia and is caused by a dominance of male hormones and can be inherited from either your father or mother. With the drop in oestrogen at the menopause the male hormones (androgens) can become more dominant, causing hair loss on the head and increased growth (and coarseness) of facial hair.

A substance called didydrotestosterone (DHT), which is made from male hormones, causes the hair to become thinner and thinner and eventually to fall out. Some women are more susceptible genetically to producing more DHT but there are steps that you can take to reduce the negative effects on your hair.

Your liver produces a protein called sex hormone-binding globulin (SHBG), which 'binds' hormones like testosterone. So if you have enough SHBG it will attach to testosterone and stop it converting to DHT.

We know that including more phytoestrogens such as soya and chickpeas (see Appendix on page 279 for a full list of phytoestrogen foods) in your diet helps your body to produce more SHBG[61] and also lignans found in flaxseeds (linseeds) stimulate the production of SHBG.[62] Eating more of these foods will help your body to control excess male hormones and stop them converting to DHT, which can affect your hair.

We also know that SHBG gets blocked by insulin so it is especially important at this stage in your life to make sure that your blood sugar is stable and not on the roller-coaster of highs and lows, causing your body to produce too much insulin.

Generally, for keeping your hair as healthy as possible, include enough protein in your diet (animal and/or vegetable) otherwise not enough can cause more hair loss. Also *don't diet*; I have seen so many women in the clinic who have gone on drastic diets and then when they go back to eating 'normally' they lose significant amounts of hair in a very short space of time because the diet is such a stress on the body. This hair loss does not happen when the women are on the diets but as soon as they stop.

SUPPLEMENTS FOR HAIR LOSS

Make sure you are taking the maintenance programme of the multivitamin and mineral designed for the menopause, Omega 3 fish oil and vitamin C. Omega 3 oils are especially important for healthy hair as they help to lubricate the hair and stop it looking dry and lifeless.

Biotin

This nutrient should be contained within your multi and is important for healthy skin and also nails. Good food sources of biotin are egg yolks, beans (soya) and pulses (lentils), brown rice and sunflower seeds. **Dose:** 25μg–1mg per day.

B vitamins

Your multi should also contain good levels of the B vitamins and these are especially important if stress has been the cause of your hair loss.
Dose: 20–25mg per day.

L-lysine

This amino acid stops testosterone from metabolising into DHT.
Dose: 300mg per day.

Saw palmetto (Serenoa repens)

This herb can be extremely helpful if you are suffering from hair loss caused by an excess of male hormones. It is usually linked to treating prostate problems because it helps to reduce the amount of DHT in the prostate but it can also be helpful for women to reduce the action of DHT on hair follicles.
Dose: 200–300mg twice daily.

Horsetail (Equisetum arvense)

This herb contains good amounts of silica, which encourages the growth of thick, healthy and shiny hair and will also help to strengthen your nails.
Dose: 300mg twice daily.

Siberian ginseng (Eleutherococcus senticosus)

This herb is especially important for you if you have been under a lot of stress and it has affected your hair.
Dose: 250–300mg twice daily.

CHAPTER 17

TESTS AND SCANS TO MONITOR YOUR ONGOING HEALTH

Testing is useful, especially when you can do something about the results. You want to be able to do a test, find out whether something is out of balance or deficient, make corrections and then retest in three months' time to make sure it is back to normal. The aim is then to maintain that for the future. It is important to correct a problem but for me the main focus is always prevention. It is much better to prevent a problem than to have to treat it.

In this chapter I will outline those tests that I think are generally useful for any woman at this stage in her life and then flag up those that are more specific to a particular problem or family history risk.

I suggest that you do whatever tests are offered as a check-up by your doctor and then add in any that need to be done privately. Some of the tests I recommend are more nutritionally orientated and will need to be done privately anyway.

An ideal scenario would be to do all the tests listed below once and then you only need to retest those that show an imbalance or deficiency. Then you may decide to have them once a year to keep on track.

GENERAL TESTS

You may be offered a blood test by your doctor that will look at your blood cells, haemoglobin and also test liver, kidney, glucose and cholesterol levels. This is a useful test to have and can highlight any problems that might need further investigation. If you are worried about hair loss then you could ask for ferritin to be measured at the same time. Faecal occult screening for colon (bowel) cancer has been introduced in the UK from the age of 60 so you will receive a kit in the post to do this test when you reach that age. You will be offered breast screening from the age of 50 and that of course is a personal choice as to what you decide to do about it (see page 243 for more information on breast screening).

There are a number of other tests that I think every woman should have from the age of 40:

- bone density scan
- bone turnover test
- vitamin D blood test
- Omega 3 to Omega 6 ratio blood test.

BONE DENSITY SCAN
This scan checks for your risk of osteoporosis and your choices as to what kind of scan you have are outlined on page 193.

BONE TURNOVER TEST
This is an extremely useful test and is done by urine testing (see page 195). It is a way of assessing whether you are losing bone on a daily basis because it is turning over (breaking down) too fast. This test is also helpful to let you know whether you are improving your bone health with your diet and supplements, because on the retest the turnover should be lower.

VITAMIN D TEST

This is a blood test and the aim is to make sure that you do not have low levels or are deficient in this important nutrient. Because research has shown that vitamin D is crucial in the prevention of cancer, especially breast cancer, heart disease, Type 2 diabetes and osteoporosis, it is important to correct a deficiency with a simple supplement of vitamin D3 and aim to maintain it.

OMEGA 3 TO OMEGA 6 RATIO BLOOD TEST

The more Omega 6 you have in your body in relation to Omega 3, the more inflammation your body is producing. We know that inflammation is implicated in so many degenerative diseases so you should aim to make sure that the balance of 3 to 6 is correct. Again it is a simple matter of taking the right supplements for a period of three months, retesting to make sure it is back to normal and then maintaining that level.

ADDITIONAL TESTS

I have listed below some extra tests that are useful if you have either a personal problem in any of these areas or a family history risk.

HEART DISEASE
Lipid blood test – cholesterol/HDL/LDL/triglycerides
I suggest that you get your cholesterol checked but also make sure that you have your HDL, LDL and triglycerides measured at the same time. This test needs to be performed on a fasting sample so make sure that you do not have anything to eat or drink (only water) after 10 p.m., ready for the blood test the next day.

C reactive protein (high sensitive) blood test
This is a marker of inflammation and is known to be important in heart disease.

Homocysteine

Higher levels of homocysteine can increase the risk of heart disease, strokes and Alzheimer's and it is easy to reduce with specific nutrients.

(See Useful Resources page 283 if you can't get these tests done locally, as many of these tests can be organised by post, or go to www.naturalhealthpractice.com.)

THE BEST BITS FOR YOU – AT A GLANCE

I'm concerned about . . .	Bone density	Bone turnover	Vitamin D	Omega 3/6	Lipids	C reactive protein	Homocysteine
My health now and keeping well	✔	✔	✔	✔	✔	✔	✔
Osteoporosis	✔	✔	✔				✔
Heart disease or strokes			✔	✔	✔	✔	✔
Alzheimer's			✔	✔		✔	✔
Breast cancer			✔	✔			

CHAPTER 18

THE GOOD NEWS

I know I have covered the doom and gloom of this stage of the menopause, offering advice on all the problems so that you can tackle them if needed, but not everyone will need it. You should know that for many women I see in the clinic, this stage can be one of the best of their lives. They are over the main menopausal symptoms (hot flushes, night sweats) or did not get them in the first place. They have the time and the energy to do what they want. Often the children have left home and they may or may not be looking after elderly parents but they are making the most of any time for themselves.

They now have another third of their life to look forward to and as Margaret Mead the famous anthropologist said, they have 'post-menopausal zest'.

These women will come into the clinic, often just once a year. They come to check that everything is staying the same nutritionally with their bone and/or heart health, for example (see recommended tests in chapter 17). For them it is like having an MOT and they want to talk over how they can keep looking after themselves, what supplements they should be taking and to focus on prevention.

It really has been 'the change' for many of these women, and often a change for the better. For some it means time to rekindle the relationship they have been in for years but the focus had been on the children and domestic pressures. For others it means the start of a new relationship or to relish time on their own, which they have never had before. We are all different and it is important to find what is important for you.

For many women I see, this stage in their life gives them the time to pursue a hobby or study a new language or even a new career. Many women have told me about taking art or music classes; either it is something they have never done before or it used to be something they enjoyed but it just got pushed aside with 'life'.

For some it is a time to travel and to see places they have not visited before and for many people in the age range 55 to 64, it can even mean taking a year out to travel. People in this age group have been termed the Golden Gappers (also known as Flash Packers). For many they just want to take enough time out to travel further afield and SKI – Spend the Kids' Inheritance. For others it can mean going to underdeveloped countries and volunteering.

The message really is to get yourself into the best of health and then maintain it so that you have the energy and the quality of life to make whatever choices you want.

APPENDIX

FOOD NUTRIENT SOURCES

Antioxidants
Apples, avocadoes, berries, broccoli, cauliflower, citrus fruits, kidney beans, nuts and seeds, oily fish, tomatoes, vegetable oils, whole grains

Beta-carotene
Butternut squash, carrots, dark green leafy vegetables, mango, papaya, peaches, peppers, sweet potato, tomatoes, watermelon

Biotin
Almonds, cabbage, cauliflower, cherries, eggs, grapefruit, herring, lettuce, oysters, peas, sweetcorn, tomatoes, watermelon

Calcium (non-dairy)
Almonds, amaranth, black beans, broccoli, brown rice, buckwheat, cabbage, chickpeas, eggs, figs, hazelnuts, parsley, pinto beans, quinoa, sardines (tinned with edible bones), Spring greens, seaweed, sesame seeds, sunflower seeds, soya, tahini, walnuts, watercress, wild salmon (tinned with edible bones)

Chromium
Apples, eggs, green peppers, oysters, parsnips, potatoes, rye

Folic acid
Asparagus, broccoli, Brussels sprouts, cashew nuts, cauliflower, sesame seeds, spinach, walnuts

Iodine
Fish, seaweed (dulse, nori, wakame)

Iron (non-meat)
Beetroot, dried apricots, molasses, parsley, prunes, pumpkin seeds, spinach, watercress

Magnesium
Apricots, broccoli, dark green leafy vegetables, figs, kale, nuts, prunes, pumpkin, sesame seeds, spinach, watercress

Manganese
Beetroot, blackberries, celery, endive, grapes, lettuce, oats, raspberries, watercress

Omega 3 (essential fatty acid)
Dark green leafy vegetables, flaxseeds (linseeds) and flaxseed oil, herring, mackerel, mustard seeds, pilchards, rapeseed oil, sardines, soya, tuna, walnuts, wild salmon

Omega 6 (essential fatty acid)
Almonds, flaxseeds (linseeds) and flaxseed oil, hemp seeds and hemp oil, pumpkin seeds, sunflower seeds, walnuts, wheat germ

Phytoestrogens
Alfalfa sprouts, chickpeas, fennel, flaxseed (linseed), lentils, miso, mung beans, parsley, sage, sesame seeds, soya milk, tamari (soy sauce), tempeh, tofu

Protein sources (non-meat)
Cheese, fish, eggs, natural yogurt, nuts and seeds, pulses, quinoa, soya milk, tofu

Selenium
Brazil nuts, brown rice, cod, molasses, oats, seafood, tuna

Superfoods
Allium family (garlic, onions, leeks and chives), apricot kernels, blueberries, broccoli, butternut squash, goji berries, pomegranate, quinoa, seaweed (dulse, nori, wakame), sprouted beans, sweet potato

Vitamin A (retinol)
Dairy produce, eggs

Vitamin B1 (Thiamin)
Asparagus, beans, Brussels sprouts, cabbage, cauliflower, courgette, lettuce, mushrooms, peas, peppers, squash, tomatoes, watercress

Vitamin B2 (Riboflavin)
Asparagus, bamboo shoots, bean sprouts, broccoli, cabbage, mackerel, mushrooms, pumpkin, tomatoes, watercress

Vitamin B3 (Niacin)
Asparagus, cabbage, courgettes, mackerel, mushrooms, salmon, squash, tomatoes, tuna

Vitamin B5 (Pantothenic acid)

Alfalfa sprouts, avocado, broccoli, cabbage, celery, eggs, lentils, mushrooms, peas, squash, strawberries, tomatoes, watercress

Vitamin B6 (Pyridoxine)

Asparagus, bananas, broccoli, Brussels sprouts, cabbage, cauliflower, kidney beans, lentils, onions, peppers, seeds and nuts, squash, watercress

Vitamin B12 (Cyanocobalamin)

Cheese, eggs, oysters, sardines, shrimp, tuna

Vitamin C

Blackcurrants, broccoli, cabbage, cauliflower, grapefruit, kiwi fruit, lemons, limes, melon, oranges, peppers, strawberries, watercress

Vitamin D

Cottage cheese, eggs, herring, mackerel, oysters, salmon

Vitamin E

Almonds, asparagus, avocado, cabbage, cashews, hazelnuts, lentils, mung beans, olive oil, olives, peas, sardines, sesame seeds, spinach, sunflower seeds, wild salmon

Zinc

Alfalfa, almonds, Brazil nuts, mung beans, oats, oysters, pecans, prawns, pumpkin seeds, sesame seeds, sunflower seeds, walnuts, wheat germ

USEFUL RESOURCES

THE DR MARILYN GLENVILLE PHD CLINICS
Consultation

All of the qualified nutritionists who work in my three UK clinics (and two in Ireland) have been trained by me in my specific approach to women's healthcare including, of course, the menopause and beyond.

Clinics are located at:

UK
- Viveka, St John's Wood, London
- The Medical Chambers, Kensington, London
- The Dr Marilyn Glenville Clinic, Tunbridge Wells, Kent.

To book a personal or telephone appointment at any of these clinics, or for more information, please contact us at:

The Dr Marilyn Glenville Clinic
14 St John's Road
Tunbridge Wells
Kent TN4 9NP
Tel: 0870 5329244/Fax: 0870 5329255
Int. Tel: +44 1 892 515905/Fax: +44 1 892 515914
Email: health@marilynglenville.com
Website: www.marilynglenville.com

Ireland

- Positive Nutrition, Dublin and Galway

To book a personal or telephone appointment at either of these clinics, or for more information, please contact us at:

Tel: 01 402 0777

Website: www.positivenutrition.ie

Supplements and tests

For more information about or to order any of the supplements and tests mentioned in this book go to:

The Natural Health Practice (NHP)

Tel: 0845 8800915

Int. Tel: + 44 1 892 507598

Website: www.naturalhealthpractice.com

The Natural Health Practice is my 'Supplier of Choice' because they stock only the highest quality, most effective nutritional supplements and natural products that have my personal approval.

Workshops and talks

For a list of my forthcoming workshops and talks, please see my website www.marilynglenville.com. If you would like me to come and give a workshop or talk near you, please call my clinic for information about how to arrange it.

Free health tips

If you would like to receive my exclusive Health Tips by email, drop me a line at health@marilynglenville.com. Just mention 'Free Health Tips' in the subject line and you will be added to my special list to receive regular health tips and other useful information.

NOTES

Chapter 1: What's going on with my hormones?

1. Rannevik, G., Jeppsson, S. and Johnell, O., 'A Longitudinal Study of the Peri-menopausal Transition: Altered Profiles of Steroid and Pituitary Hormones, SHBG and Bone Mineral Density', *Maturitas,* **8** (1986), 189–96

Chapter 2: My Twelve-Step Hormone Balancing Diet

1. Colomer, R. and Menendez, J.A., 'Mediterranean Diet, Olive Oil and Cancer', *Clin Transl Oncol*, **8** (2006), 15–21
2. Ta, M.H., Xu, W.H., Zheng, W. *et al.*, 'A Case-controlled Study in Shanghai of Fruit and Vegetable Intake and Endometrial Cancer', *Br J Cancer*, **92** (2005), 2059–64
3. Kiania, F., Knutsen, S., Singh, P. *et al.*, 'Dietary Risk Factors for Ovarian Cancer: The Adventist Health Study (US)', *Cancer Causes Control*, **17** (2006), 137–46
4. Nagata, C. *et al.*, 'Soy Product Intake and Hot Flushes in Japanese Women: Results from a Community Based Prospective Study', *Am J Epidem*, **153** (2001), 790–3
5. Martinez, M.E. *et al.*, 'Soy and Breast Cancer: The Controversy Continues', *J Natl Cancer Inst*, **98** (2006), 430–1
6. Qin, L.Q. *et al.*, 'Soyfood Intake in the Prevention of Breast Cancer Risk in Women: A Meta-Analysis of Observational Epidemiological Studies', *J Nutr Sci Vitaminol (Tokyo)*, **52** (2006), 6, 428–36
7. Dhom, G., 'Epidemiology of Hormone Dependent Tumours', in *Endocrine Dependent Tumours* (K.D. Voigt and C. Knabbe, eds.) (1991), Raven Press, New York
8. Griffiths, K., 'Oestrogen and Prostatic Disease', International Prostate Health Study Group, *Prostate*, **45** (2000), 2, 87–100
9. Haggans, C.J. *et al.*, 'The Effect of Flaxseed Consumption on Urinary Estrogen Metabolites in Premenopausal Women', *Cancer Epid Bio Prev*, **9** (2000), 719–25
10. Simopoulos, A.O., 'Omega-3 Fatty Acids in Health and Disease and in Growth and Development', *Am J Clin Nutr*, **54** (1991), 438–63
11. Nagata, C., Takatsuka, N., Kawakami, N. *et al.*, 'Total and Monounsaturated Fat Intake and Serum Estrogen Concentrations in Premenopausal Japanese Women', *Nutr Cancer*, **38** (2000), 37–9

12. de Roos, N.M. *et al.*, 'Trans Fatty Acids, HDL-cholesterol, and Cardiovascular Disease. Effects of Dietary Changes on Vascular Reactivity', *Eur J Med Res*, **8** (2003), 8, 355–7

13. Theodore, R.F. *et al.*, 'Dietary Patterns and Intelligence in Early and Middle Childhood', *Intelligence*, **37** (2009), 506–13

14. Blundell, J.E. and Hill, A.J., 'Paradoxical Effects of an Intense Sweetener (Aspartame) on Appetite', *Lancet*, **1** (1986), 8489, 1092–3

15. Haggans, C.J. *et al.*, 'The Effect of Flaxseed and Wheat Bran Consumption on Urinary Estrogen Metabolites in Premenopausal Women', *Cancer Epid Bio Prev*, **9** (2000), 719–25

16. Barton, L., 'A Spoonful of Propaganda', *Guardian*, Friday 12 April 2002

17. COI Communications and the Food Standards Agency, 'Investigation of consumer understanding of sugars labelling on front of pack nutritional signposts, without specific reference to breakfast cereals', COI Ref. 279259

18. Welsh, J.A. *et al.*, 'Caloric Sweetener Consumption and Dyslipidemia among US Adults', *JAMA*, **303** (2010), 15, 1490–7

19. Bolland, M.J. *et al.*, 'Effect of Calcium Supplements on Risk of Myocardial Infarction and Cardiovascular Events: Meta-analysis', *BMJ*, **341** (2010), 3691

20. Sakhaee, K. *et al.*, 'A Meta-analysis of Calcium Bioavailability: A Comparison of Calcium Citrate with Calcium Carbonate', *American Journal of Therapeutics*, **5** (1999), 313–21

21. Trang, H.M. *et al.*, 'Evidence that Vitamin D3 Increases Serum 25-hydroxyvitamin D More Efficiently than does Vitamin D2', *Am J Clin Nutr*, **68** (1998), 854–8

Chapter 3: Exercise – for today and tomorrow

1. Chang, H.J., Lynm, C. and Glass, R.M., 'Hypertrophic Cardiomyopathy', *JAMA*, **302** (2009), 15, 1720

2. Lahmann, P.H. *et al.*, 'Physical Activity and Breast Cancer Risk: The European Prospective Investigation into Cancer and Nutrition', *Cancer Epid Bio Prev*, **16** (2007), 36–42

3. McGuire, K.A. *et al.*, 'Ability of Physical Activity to Predict Cardiovascular Disease beyond Commonly Evaluated Cardiometabolic Risk Factors', *Am J Cardio*, **104** (2009), 11, 152–6

4. Leon, A.S. and Sanchez, O.A., 'Response of Blood Lipids to Exercise Training Alone or Combined with Dietary Intervention', *Med Sci Sports Exerc*, **33** (2001), 6, S502–15

5. Beavers, K.M., 'Effect of Exercise Training on Chronic Inflammation', *Clin Chim Acta*, 25 Feb 2010

6. Thomas, D.E. *et al.*, 'Exercise for Type 2 Diabetes Mellitus', *Cochrane Database Syst Rev*, **19** (2006), 3, CD002968

7. Haaland, D.A. *et al.*, 'Is Regular Exercise a Friend or Foe of the Ageing Immune System? A Systematic Review', *Clin J Sport Med*, **18** (2008), 6, 539–48

8. Chubak, J., 'Moderate-intensity Exercise Reduces the Incidence of Colds in Postmenopausal Women', *Am J Med*, **119** (2006), 11, 937–42

9. Cherkas, L.F. *et al.*, 'The Association Between Physical Activity in Leisure Time and Leukocyte Telomere Length', *Arch Intern Med*, **168** (2008), 2, 154–8

10. Suzuki, S. *et al.*, 'Effect of Physical Activity on Breast Cancer Risk: Findings of the Japan Collaborative Cohort Study', *Cancer Epid Bio Prev*, **17** (2008), 12, 3396–401

11. Wolin, K.Y. *et al.*, 'Physical Activity and Colon Cancer Prevention: A Meta–analysis', *Br J Cancer*, **100** (2009), 4, 611–16

12. Tenenbaum, G., 'The Effect of Music Type on Running Perseverance and Coping with Effort Sensations', *Psychology of Sport and Exercise*, **5** (2004), 2, 89–109

Chapter 4: Anti-ageing and how to slow down the clock

1. Lee, S.J. *et al.,* 'Spoonful of Sugar Makes the Worms' Life Span go Down', *Science Daily*, Cell Press, 5 November 2009

2. Kiecolt-Glaser, J.K. *et al.*, 'Depressive Symptoms, Omega 3: Omega 6 Fatty Acids and Inflammation in Older Adults', *Psychom Med*, **69** (2007), 3, 217–24

3. Schaefer, E.J. *et al.,* 'Plasma Phosphatidylcholine docosahexaenoic Acid Content and Risk of Dementia and Alzheimer Disease: The Framingham Heart Study', *Arch Neurol*, **63** (2006), 11, 1545–50

4. Ma, Q.L. *et al.*, 'Omega 3 Fatty Acid Docosahexaenoic Acid Increases SorLA/LR11, a Sorting Protein with Reduced Expression in Sporadic Alzheimer's Disease (AD): Relevance to AD Prevention', *J Neurosci*, **27** (2007), 52, 14299–307

5. Epel, E.S. *et al.*, 'Accelerated Telomere Shortening in Response to Life Stress', *Proc Nat Acad Sci*, **101** (2004), 49, 17312–15

6. Srinivasan, V. *et al.*, 'Melatonin, Immune Function and Ageing', *Immunity & Ageing*, **2** (2005), 17

7. Nowson, C.A. and Magerison, C., 'Vitamin D Intake and Vitamin D Status of Australians', *Med J Aust*, **177** (2002), 3, 149–52

8. Richards, J.B. *et al.*, 'Higher Serum Vitamin D Concentrations are Associated with Longer Leukocyte Telomere Length in Women', *Am J Clin Nutr*, **86** (2007), 5, 1420–5

9. Fontana, L. *et al.*, Long-term Low-protein, Low-calorie Diet and Endurance Exercise Modulate Metabolic Factors Associated with Cancer Risk', *Am J Clin Nutr*, **4** (2006), 6, 456–62

10. Singh, R.B. *et al.*, 'Effect of Hydrosoluble Coenzyme Q10 on Blood Pressures and Insulin Resistance in Hypertensive Patients with Coronary Artery Disease', *J Hum Hypertens*, **13** (1999), 203–8

11. Wolfram, S. *et al.*, 'Anti-obesity Effects of Green Tea: From Bedside to Bench', *Mol Nutr Food Res*, **50** (2006), 2, 176–87

Chapter 5: Lifestyle changes

1. Tasali, E. *et al.,* 'Slow Wave Sleep and the Risk of Type 2 Diabetes in Humans', *Proc Natl Acad Sci*, **105** (2008), 3, 1044–9

2. Shakhar, K. *et al.*, 'Sleep, Fatigue and NK Cell Activity in Healthy Volunteers: Significant Relationships Revealed within Subject Analyses', *Brain, Behaviour and Immunity*, **21** (2007), 2, 180–4

3. Patel, S.R. *et al.*, 'Association Between Reduced Sleep and Weight Gain in Women', *Am J Epidemiol*, **164** (2006), 10, 947–54

4. Melzer, D. *et al.*, 'Association Between Serum Perfluoroctanoic Acid (PFOA) and Thyroid Disease in the NHANES Study', *Environ Health Perspect*, 7 Jan 2010

5. Gibbons, A., 'Dioxin Tied to Endometriosis', *Science*, **262** (1993), 1373

Chapter 6: Have you started to go through the menopause?

1. Siddle, N. *et al.*, 'The Effect of Hysterectomy on the Age of Ovarian Failure: Identification of a Subgroup of Women with Premature Loss of Ovarian Function and Literature Review', *Fertility and Sterility*, **47** (1987), 1, 94–100

2. Turney, L., 'Risk and Contraception: What Women are not Told about Tubal Ligation', *Women's Studies International Forum*, **16** (1993), 5, 471–86

3. Soules, M.R., Sherman, S., Parrott, E. *et al.*, 'Executive Summary: Stages of Reproductive Aging Workshop (STRAW)' *Fertility and Sterility*, **5** (2001), 874–8

4. Research presented at the European Society of Human Reproduction and Embryology conference in 2010

5. Lindenbaum, J. *et al.*, 'Oral Contraceptive Hormones, Folate, Metabolism and the Cervical Epithelium', *Am Jo Clin Nutr*, **28** (1975), 4, 346–53

6. Van Niekerk, W., 'Cervical Cytological Abnormalities Caused by Folic Acid Deficiency', *Acta Cytol*, **10** (1966), 67–73

7. Whitehead, N. *et al.*, 'Megaloblastic Changes in the Cervical Epithelium: Association with Oral Contraceptive Therapy and Reversal with Folic Acid', *JAMA*, **226** (1973), 1421–4

8. Hernandez, B.Y., McDuffie, K., Wilkens, L.R. *et al.*, 'Diet and Premalignant Lesions of the Cervix: Evidence of a Protective Role for Folate, Riboflavin, Thiamin and Vitamin B12', *Cancer Causes Control*, **14** (2003), 9, 859–70

9. Smith, J.S., Green, J., Berrington de Gonzalez, A. *et al.*, 'Cervical Cancer and Use of Hormonal Contraceptives: A Systemic Review', *Lancet*, **361** (2003), 1159–63

10. Kahlenborn, C. *et al.*, 'Oral Contraceptive Use as a Risk Factor for Premenopausal Breast Cancer: A Meta-Analysis', *Mayo Clin Proc*, **81** (2006), 1287–9

11. Anderson, K. and Rybo, G., 'Levonorgestrel-releasing Uterine Device in the Treatment of Menorrhagia', *Br J Obstet Gynaecol*, **97** (1990), 690–4

Chapter 7: What to eat and what to avoid

1. Nagata, C. *et al.*, 'Soy Product Intake and Hot Flashes in Japanese Women: Results from a Community-based Prospective Study', *Am J Epidem*, **153** (2001), 8, 790–3

Chapter 8: How supplements and herbs can help you

1. Lucas, M. *et al.*, 'Effects of EPA Omega 3 Fatty Acid Supplementation on Hot Flashes and Quality of Life Among Middle Aged Women: A Double Blind, Placebo Controlled, Randomised Clinical Trial', *Menopause*, **16** (2009), 2, 357–66

2. Hassan, I. *et al.*, 'PMS in the Perimenopause', *J Brit Meno Soc*, **10** (2004), 4, 151–6

3. Di Carlo, C. *et al.*, 'Use of Leuprolide Acetate Plus Tibolone in the Treatment of Severe Premenstrual Syndrome', *Fertil Steril*, **75** (2001), 380–4

4. Hassan, I. *et al.*, 'PMS in the Perimenopause', *J Brit Meno Soc*, **10** (2004), 4, 151–6

5. Rubinow, D.H. *et al.*, 'Changes in Plasma Hormones across the Menstrual Cycle in Patients with Menstrually Related Mood Disorder', *Am J Obstet Gynecol*, **158** (1988), 5–11

6. Schmidt, P.J. *et al.*, 'Differential Behavioural Effects of Gonadal Steroids in Women with and in those Without Pre-menstrual Syndrome', *NEJM*, **338** (1998), 4, 209–16

7. Schellenberg, R., 'A Good Double Blind Placebo Controlled Clinical Trial in the *British Medical Journal* Showed that Agnus Castus is an 'effective and well tolerated treatment' for PMS', *BMJ*, **322** (2001), 134–7

8. Atmaca, M. *et al.*, 'Fluoxetine versus *Vitex Agnus Castus* Extract in the Treatment of Premenstrual Dysphoric Disorder', *Hum Psychopharmacol*, **18** (2003), 3, 191–5

9. Low Dog, T., 'Menopause: A Review of Botanical Dietary Supplements', *Am J Med*, **118** (2005), Suppl 12B, 98–108

10. Geller, S.E. and Studee, L., 'Botanical and Dietary Supplements for Mood and Anxiety in Menopausal Women', *Menopause*, **14** (2007), 3, 541–9

11. Reed, S.D. *et al.*, 'Vaginal, Endometrial and Reproductive Hormone Findings: Randomised Placebo-controlled Trial of Black Cohosh, Multibotanical Herbs and Dietary Soy for Vasomotor Symptoms: The Herbal Alternatives for Menopause (HALT) Study', *Menopause*, **15** (2008), 1, 51–8

12. Liske, E. *et al.*, 'Physiological Investigation of a Unique Extract of Black Cohosh (*Cimicifugae Racemosae Rhizoma*): A 6-month Clinical Study Demonstrates no Systemic Estrogenic Effect', *J Womens Health Gend Based Med*, **11** (2002), 2, 163–74

13. Al-Akoum, M. *et al.*, 'Synergistic Cytotoxic Effects of Tamoxifen and Black Cohosh on MCF-7 and MDA-MB-231 Human Breast Cancer Cells: An In Vitro Study', *Can J Physiol Pharmacol*, **85** (2007), 11, 1153–9

14. Rebbeck, T.R. and Troxel, A.B., 'A Retrospective Case-control Study of the Use of Hormone-related Supplements and Association with Breast Cancer', *Int J Cancer*, **120** (2007), 7, 1523–8

15. Bodinet, C. and Freudenstein, J., 'Influence of *Cimicifuga Racemosa* on the Proliferation of Estrogen Receptor-positive Human Breast Cancer Cells', *Breast Cancer Res Treat*, **76** (2002), 1–10

16. Kupfersztain, C. *et al.*, 'The Immediate Effect of Natural Plant Extract, *Angelica Sinensis* and *Matricaria Chamomilla* (Climex) for the Treatment of Hot Flushes During the Menopause: A Preliminary Report', *Clin Exp Obstet Gynecol*, **30** (2003), 4, 203–6

17. De Leo, V. *et al.*, 'Treatment of Neurovegetative Menopausal Symptoms with a Phytotherapeutic Agent', *Minerva Ginecol*, **50** (1998), 207–11

18. Woelk, H., 'Comparison of St John's Wort and Imipramine for Treating Depression: Randomised Controlled Trial', *BMJ*, **313** (2000), 253–61

19. Al-Akoum, M. *et al.*, 'Effects of *Hypericum Perforatum* (St John's Wort) on Hot Flashes and Quality of Life in Perimenopausal Women: A Randomised Pilot Trial', *Menopause*, **16** (2009), 2, 307–14

Chapter 9: Keep moving

1. Daley, A.J. and Stokes-Lampard, H.J., 'Exercise to Reduce Vasomotor and Other Menopausal Symptoms: A Review', *Maturitas*, **20** (2009), 63, 176–80

2. McAndrew, L.M. *et al.*, 'When, Why and for Whom there is a Relationship Between Physical Activity and Menopause Symptoms', *Maturitas*, **20** (2009), 64, 2, 119–25
3. Yaffe, K., 'A Prospective Study of Physical Activity and Cognitive Decline in Elderly Women: Women who Walk', *Arch Intern Med*, **161** (2001), 14, 1703–8
4. Rovio, S. *et al.*, 'Leisure Time Physical Activity at Midlife and the Risk of Dementia and Alzheimer's Disease', *Lancet Neurol*, **4** (2005), 11, 705–11
5. Richards, M. *et al.*, 'Does Active Leisure Protect Cognition? Evidence from a National Birth Cohort', *Soc Sci Med*, **56** (2003), 785–92
6. Schmitz, K.H., 'Strength Training and Adiposity in Premenopausal Women: Strong, Healthy and Empowered Study', *Am J Clin Nutr*, **86** (2007), 3, 566–72
7. Fred Hutchinson Cancer Research Center, 'Regular Yoga Practice may Help Prevent Middle-age Spread', *Science Daily*, 21 July 2005
8. Presented at The Endocrine Society's 90th Annual Meeting in San Francisco
9. Hourigan, S.R. *et al.*, 'Positive Effects of Exercise on Falls and Fracture Risk in Osteopenic Women', *Osteoporosis*, **19** (2008), 7, 1077–86
10. Lindau, S.T. and Gavrilova, N., 'Sex, Health and Years of Sexually Active Life Gained due to Good Health: Evidence from Two US Population Based Cross Sectional Surveys of Ageing', *BMJ*, **340** (2010), 810

Chapter 10: How to control your weight

1. World Cancer Research Fund report 'Food, Nutrition, Physical Activity and the Prevention of Cancer' (2007)
2. Gonzalez, E.L. *et al.*, 'Trends in the Prevalence and Incidence of Diabetes in the UK: 1996–2005', *Journal of Epidemiology and Community Health*, **63** (2009), 4, 332–6
3. WHO report (October 2005)
4. Hession, M. *et al.*, 'Systematic Review of Randomized Controlled Trials of Low-carbohydrate vs. Low-fat/Low-calorie Diets in the Management of Obesity and its Comorbidities, *Obes Rev*, **10** (2009), 1, 36–50
5. Balk, E.M. *et al.*, 'Effect of Chromium Supplementation on Glucose Metabolism and Lipids: A Systematic Review of Randomised Controlled Trials', *Diabetes Care*, **30** (2007), 8, 2154–63
6. Nahas, R. and Moher, M., 'Complementary and Alternative Medicine for the Treatment of Type 2 Diabetes', *Can Fam Physician*, **55** (2009), 6, 591–6
7. Kao, W.H. *et al.*, 'Serum and Dietary Magnesium and the Risk for Type 2 Diabetes Mellitus: The Atherosclerosis Risk in Communities Study', *Arch Intern Med*, **159** (1999), 18, 2151–9
8. Chen, M.D. *et al.*, 'Zinc May be a Mediator of Leptin Production in Humans', *Life Sci*, **66** (2000), 22, 2143–9
9. Ford, E.S. *et al.*, 'The Metabolic Syndrome and Antioxidant Concentrations: Findings from the Third National Health and Nutrition Examination Survey', *Diabetes*, **52** (2003), 9, 2346–52
10. Chen, L. and Thacker, R., 'Effects of Dietary Vitamin E and High Supplementation of Vitamin C on Plasma Glucose and Cholesterol Levels', *Nutr Res*, **5** (1985), 527–34

11. Johnston, C.S., 'Strategies for Healthy Weight Loss: From Vitamin C to the Glycemic Response', *J Am Coll Nutr*, **24** (2005), 158–65

12. Souza, L.L., Nunes, M.O., Paula, G.S. *et al.*, 'Effects of Dietary Fish Oil on Thyroid Hormone Signalling in the Liver', *J Nutr Biochem*, 28 Sep 2009

13. Mu Li *et al.*, 'Declining Iodine Content of Milk and Re-emergence of Iodine Deficiency in Australia', *MJA*, **184** (2006), 6, 307

Chapter 11: HRT and bioidentical hormones

1. Writing Group for the Women's Health Initiative Investigators, 'Risks and Benefits of Estrogen Plus Progestin in Healthy Postmenopausal Women', *JAMA*, **288** (2002), 321–33

2. Million Women Study Collaborators, 'Breast Cancer and Hormone Replacement Therapy in the Million Women Study', *Lancet*, **362** (2003), 419–27

3. Studd, J., 'Why are Physicians Reluctant to Use Oestrogens for Anything – or Do They Prefer "PROFOX"?', *Meno Int*, **15** (2009), 52–4

4. Whitehead, M. and Farmer, R., 'The Million Women Study: A Critique', *Endocrine*, **24** (2004), 187–94

5. Marsden, J. and Sturdee, D., 'Cancer Issue', *Best Pract Res Clin Obstet Gynaecol*, **23** (2009), 87–107

6. Rosendaal, F.R., 'Hormone Replacement Therapy and Thrombotic Risk: Beauty is only Skin Deep', *Nat Clin Pract Cardiovasc Med*, **5** (2008), 11, 684–5

7. Chlebowski, R.T. *et al.*, 'Breast Cancer after Use of Oestrogen Plus Progestin in Post-menopausal Women', *NEJM*, **360** (2009), 573–87

8. Brown, S., 'More Reports Link Falling Breast Cancer Rates to Change in Use of Hormone Replacement Therapy', *Meno Int*, **15** (2009), 48–9

9. Parkin, D.M., 'Is the Recent Fall in Incidence of Post-menopausal Breast Cancer in UK Related to Changes in Use of Hormone Replacement Therapy?', *Eur J Cancer*, **45** (2009), 1649–53

10. Heiss, G. *et al.*, 'Health Risks and Benefits 3 Years after Stopping Randomised Treatment with Oestrogen and Progestin', *JAMA*, **299** (2008), 1036–45

11. Liu, B. *et al.*, 'Reproductive History, Hormonal Factors and the Incidence of Hip and Knee Replacement for Osteoarthritis in Middle Aged Women', *Ann Rheum Dis*, **68** (2009), 1165–70

12. Hays, J. *et al.*, 'Effects of Estrogen plus Progestin on Health-related Quality of Life', *NEJM*, **348** (2003), 19, 1835–7

13. EMEA, 'Further Advice on Safety of Hormone Replacement Therapy: No Longer Recommended as First Choice for Prevention of Osteoporosis', *HMA* (www.hma.eu/uploads)

14. Heikkinen, J. *et al.*, 'A 10 Year Follow Up of the effect of Continuous Combined Hormone Replacement Therapy and its Discontinuation on Bone in Postmenopausal Women', *Meno Int*, **14** (2008), 70–7

15. Craig, M.C. *et al.*, 'The Women's Health Initiative Memory Study: Findings and Implications for Treatment', *Lancet Neurol*, **4** (2005), 3, 190–4

16. Grady, D. *et al.*, 'Postmenopausal Hormones and Incontinence: The Heart and Estrogen/Progestin Replacement Study', *Obstetrics and Gynaecology*, **97** (2001), 116–20
17. Holtorf, K., 'The Bioidentical Hormone Debate: Are Bioidentical Hormones (Oestradiol, Estriol and Progesterone) Safer or More Efficacious than Commonly Used Synthetic Versions in Hormone Replacement Therapy?', *Postgrad Med*, **121** (2009), 1, 73–85
18. Boothby, L.A. and Doering, P.L., 'Bioidentical Hormone Therapy: A Panacea that Lacks Supportive Evidence', *Curr Opin Obstet Gynecol*, **20** (2008), 4, 400–7
19. FDA Consumer Health Information Leaflet, 'Bioidenticals – Sorting Myths from Facts', www.fda.gov/consumer/updates/bioidenticals040808.html
20. Eden, J.A., Hacker, N.F. and Fortune, M., 'Three Cases of Endometrial Cancer Associated with "Bioidentical" Hormone Replacement Therapy', *Med J of Aust*, **187** (2007), 4, 244–5
21. Soares, R. *et al.*, 'Elucidating Progesterone Effects in Breast Cancer: Cross Talk with PDGF Signalling Pathway in Smooth Muscle Cell', *J Cell Biochem*, **100** (2007), 174–83
22. Carvajal, A., 'Progesterone Pre-treatment Potentiates EGF Pathway Signaling in the Breast Cancer Cell Line ZR-75', *Breast Cancer Res Treat*, **94** (2005), 171–83
23. Benster, B. *et al.*, 'Double Blind Placebo-controlled Study to Evaluate the Effect of Pro-juven Progesterone Cream on Atherosclerosis and Bone Density', *Meno Int*, **15** (2009), 100–1
24. Benster, B. *et al.*, 'A Double-blind Placebo-controlled Study to Evaluate the Effect of Progestelle Progesterone Cream on Postmenopausal Women', *Meno Int*, **15** (2009), 63–9

Chapter 12: Tests and scans
1. Stewart, A. *et al.*, 'Long Term Fracture Prediction by DXA and QUS: A 10 Year Prospective Study', *J Bone Miner Res*, **21** (2006), 413–18
2. Ganero, P., 'Biomarkers for Osteoporosis Management: Utility in Diagnosis, Fracture Risk Prediction and Therapy Monitoring', *Mol Diagn Ther*, **12** (2008), 3, 157–70
3. Eastell, R. and Hannon, R.A., 'Biomarkers of Bone Health and Osteoporosis Risk', *Proc Nutr Soc*, **67** (2008), 2, 157–62

Chapter 14: Your diet, food supplements and exercise
1. Eastell, R. and Hannon, R.A., 'Biomarkers of Bone Health and Osteoporosis Risk', *Proc Nutr Soc*, **67** (2008), 2, 157–62
2. Koh, W.P. *et al.*, 'Gender-specific Associations Between Soy and risk of Hip Fracture in the Singapore Chinese Health Study', *Am J Epidemiol*, **170** (2009), 7, 901–9
3. Stephens, N.G. *et al.*, 'Randomised controlled trial of vitamin E in patients with coronary disease: Cambridge Heart Antioxidant Study (CHAOS)', *Lancet*, **347** (1996), 9004, 78–6
4. McLean, R.R. *et al.*, 'Plasma B Vitamins, Homocysteine, and their Relation with Bone Loss and Hip Fracture in Elderly Men and Women', *J Clin Endocrinol Metab*, **93** (2008), 6, 2206–12
5. Requirand, P. *et al.*, 'Serum Fatty Acid Imbalance in Bone Loss: Example with Periodontal Disease', *Clin Nutr*, **19** (2000), 4, 271–6

6. Lavie, C., 'Omega 3 Polyunsaturated Fatty Acids and Cardiovascular Diseases', *Journal of the American College of Cardiology*, **54** (2009), 7, 585–94

7. Danaei, G. *et al.*, 'The Preventable Causes of Death in the United States: Comparative Risk Assessment of Dietary, Lifestyle, and Metabolic Risk Factors', study, April 2009, *PLoS Medicine*

8. Sahni, S. *et al.*, 'Protective Effect of Total and Supplemental Vitamin C intake on the Risk of Hip Fracture – 17 Year Follow Up from the Framingham Osteoporosis Study', *Osteoporosis Int*, **20** (2009), 11, 1853–61

9. Beavers, K.M., 'Effect of Exercise Training on Chronic Inflammation', *Clin Chim Acta*, 25 Feb 2010

10. Hourigan, S. *et al.*, 'Positive Effects of Exercise on Falls and Fracture Risk on Osteopenic Women', *Osteoporosis Int*, **19** (2008), 7, 1077–86

Chapter 15: Osteoporosis – how to prevent, stop and even reverse it

1. Frassetto, L.A. *et al.*, 'Worldwide Incidence of Hip Fractures in Elderly Women: Relation to Consumption of Animal and Vegetable Foods', *J Gerontol A Biol Sci Med Sci*, **55** (2000), 10, M585–92

2. Lanham-New, S.A., 'Fruit and Vegetables: The Unexpected Natural Answer to the Question of Osteoporosis Prevention?', *Am J Clin Nutr*, **83** (2006), 6, 1254–5

3. Weikert, C. *et al.*, 'The Relation Between Dietary Protein, Calcium and Bone Health in Women: Results from the EPIC-Potsdam Cohort', *Ann Nutr Metab*, **49** (2005), 5, 312–18

4. Sellmeyer, D.E. *et al.*, 'A High Ratio of Dietary Animal to Vegetable Protein Increases the Rate of Bone Loss and the Risk of Fracture in Postmenopausal Women', *Am J Clin Nutr*, **73** (2001), 1, 118–22

5. Remer, T. and Manz, F., 'Potential Renal Acid Load of Foods and its Influence on Urine pH', *J Am Diet Assoc*, **95** (1995), 791–7

6. Tucker, K.L. *et al.*, 'Colas, but Not Other Carbonated Beverages, are Associated with Low Bone Mineral Density in Older Women: The Framingham Osteoporosis Study', **84** (2006), 4, 936–42

7. Welch, A.A. *et al.*, 'Urine pH is an Indicator of Dietary Acid-base Load, Fruit and Vegetables and Meat Intakes: Results from the European Prospective Investigation into Cancer and Nutrition (EPIC) Norfolk Population Study', *Br J Nutr*, **99** (2008), 6, 1335–43

8. Goodman, G.D., 'Interleukin-6: An Osteotropic Factor?', *J Bone Miner Res*, 7 (1992), 475–6

9. Fernandes, G. *et al.*, 'Effects of Omega 3 Fatty Acids on Autoimmunity and Osteoporosis', *Front Biosci*, **1** (2008), 13, 4015–20

10. Gjesdal, C.G. *et al.*, 'Plasma Homocysteine, Folate and Vitamin B12 and the Risk of Hip Fracture: The Hordaland Homocysteine Study', **22** (2007), 747–56

11. Lean, J.M. *et al.*, 'A Crucial Role for Thiol Antioxidants in Oestrogen Deficiency Bone Loss', *J Clin Invest*, **112** (2003), 6, 915–23

12. Sugiura, M. *et al.*, 'Bone Mineral Density in Postmenopausal Female Subjects is Associated with Serum Antioxidant Carotenoids', *Osteoporosis Int*, **19** (2008), 2, 211–19

13. Matheson, E.M. *et al.*, 'The Association Between Onion Consumption and Bone Density in Perimenopausal and Postmenopausal Non-Hispanic White Women 50 Years and Older', *Menopause*, **16** (2009), 4, 756–9

14. Feskanich, D. *et al.*, 'Vitamin K Intake and Hip Fractures in Women: A Prospective Study', *Am J Clin Nutr*, **69** (1999), 1, 74–9

15. Iwamoto, J., 'High Dose Vitamin K Supplementation Reduces Fracture Indices in Postmenopausal Women: A Review of the Literature', *Nutr Res*, **29** (2009), 4, 221–8

16. Elia, M. and Cummings, J.H., 'Physiological Aspects of Energy Metabolism and Gastrointestinal Effects of Carbohydrates', *Eur J Clin Nutri*, **61** (2007), Suppl 1, 40–74

17. Shea, B. *et al.*, 'Role of Calcium in Reducing Postmenopausal Bone Loss and in Fracture Prevention', *Endocrine Rev*, **23** (2002), 4, 522–9

18. Shea, B. *et al.*, 'Calcium Supplementation on Bone Loss in Postmenopausal Women', *Cochrane Database Syst Rev*, **1** (2004), CD004526

19. Ensrud, K.E. *et al.*, 'Effects of Raloxifene on Fracture Risk in Postmenopausal Women: The Raloxifene Use for the Heart Trial', *J Bone Miner Res*, **23** (2008), 1, 112–20

20. Wells, G.A. *et al.*, 'Alendronate for the Primary and Secondary Prevention of Osteoporotic Fractures in Postmenopausal Women', *Cochrane Database Syst Rev*, **1** (2008), CD001155

21. Tonino, R.P. *et al.*, 'Skeletal Benefits of Alendronate Seven Year Treatment of Postmenopausal Osteoporotic Women', *J Clin Endocrinol Metabol*, **85** (2000), 3109–15

22. Presented at the 2010 Annual Meeting of the American Academy of Orthopaedic Surgeons

23. Watts, N.B. and Diab, D.L., 'Long Term Use of Bisphosphonates in Osteoporosis', *J Clin Endocrinol Metab*, **95** (2010), 4, 1555–65

24. Alonso-Coello, P. *et al.*, 'Drugs for Pre-osteoporosis: Prevention or Disease Mongering?', *BMJ*, **336** (2008), 126–9

25. Meunier, P.J., 'The Effects of Strontium Ranelate on the Risk of Vertebral Fracture in Women with Postmenopausal Osteoporosis', *NEJM*, **350** (2004), 459–68

26. Neer, R.M., 'Effect of Parathyroid Hormone (1-34) on Fractures and Bone Mineral Density in Postmenopausal Women with Osteoporosis', *NEJM*, **344** (2001), 1434–41

27. Cummings, S.R. *et al.*, 'Denosumab for Prevention of Fractures in Postmenopausal Women with Osteoporosis', *NEJM*, **361** (2009), 8, 756–65

Chapter 16: Other health risks after the menopause

1. Howard, B.V. *et al.*, 'Low-fat Dietary Pattern and Risk of Cardiovascular Disease: The Women's Health Initiative Randomized Controlled Dietary Modification Trial', *JAMA*, **295** (2006), 6, 655-66 and Prentice, R.L. *et al.*, 'Low-fat Dietary Pattern and Risk of Invasive Breast Cancer: The Women's Health Initiative Randomized Controlled Dietary Modification Trial', *JAMA*, **295** (2006), 6, 629–42

2. Siri-Tarino, P.W. *et al.*, 'Meta-analysis of Prospective Cohort Studies Evaluating the Association of Saturated Fat with Cardiovascular Disease', *Am J Clin Nutr*, **91** (2010), 3, 535–46

3. Hession, M. *et al.*, 'Systematic Review of Randomized Controlled Trials of Low-carbohydrate vs. Low-fat/Low-calorie Diets in the Management of Obesity and its Comorbidities', *Obes Rev*, **10** (2009), 1, 36–50

4. Sachdeva, A. *et al.*, 'Lipid Levels in Patients Hospitalized with Coronary Artery Disease: An Analysis of 136,905 Hospitalizations in Get With the Guidelines', *Am Heart J*, **57** (2009), 111–7

5. Al-Mallah, M.H. *et al.*, 'Low Admission LDL-cholesterol is Associated with Increased 3-year All-cause Mortality in Patients with Non ST Segment Elevation Myocardial Infarction', *Cardiol J*, **16** (2009), 227–33

6. Rossebo, A.B. *et al.*, 'Intensive Lipid Lowering with Simvastin and Ezetimibe in Aortic Stenosis', *NEJM*, **359** (2008), 13, 1343–56

7. de Lorgeril, M. *et al.*, 'Mediterranean Diet, Traditional Risk Factors and the Rate of Cardiovascular Complication after Myocardial Infarction: Final Report of the Lyon Diet Heart Study', *Circulation*, **99** (1999), 779–85

8. Walsh, J.M.E. *et al.*, 'Drug Treatment of Hyperlipidemia in Women', *JAMA*, **291** (2004), 2243–52

9. Hodis, H.N. and Mack, W.J., 'Postmenopausal Hormone Therapy in Clinical Perspective', *Menopause*, **14** (2007), 1–14

10. Berger, J.S. *et al.*, 'Aspirin for the Primary Prevention of Cardiovascular Events in Women and Men: A Sex Specific Meta-analysis of Randomized Controlled Trials', *JAMA*, **295** (2006), 306–13

11. Rundek, T. *et al.*, 'Atorvastin Decreases the Coenzyme Q10 Level in the Blood of Patients at Risk of Cardiovascular Disease and Stroke', *Arch Neurol*, **61** (2004), 6, 889–92

12. Singh, R.B. *et al.*, 'Effect of Hydrosoluble Coenzyme Q10 on Blood Pressures and Insulin Resistance in Hypertensive Patients with Coronary Artery Disease', *J Hum Hypertens*, **13** (1999), 203–8

13. Ascer, E. *et al.*, 'Atorvastatin Reduces Proinflammatory Markers in Hypercholesterolemic Patients', *Atherosclerosis*, **177** (2004), 1, 161–6

14. Pfleilschifler, J. *et al.*, 'Changes in Pro-inflammatory Cytokine Activity after Menopause', *Endocrine Reviews*, **23** (2002), 90

15. Jupiter Study, presented at the American Heart Association's scientific meeting in 2009

16. Setola, E. *et al.*, 'Insulin Resistance and Endothelial Function are Improved After Folate and Vitamin B12 Therapy in Patients with Metabolic Syndrome: Relationship Between Homocysteine levels and Hyperinsulinemia', *Eur J Endocrinol*, **15** (2004), 4, 483–9

17. Van den Berghe, G. *et al.*, 'Bone Turnover in Prolonged Critical Illness: Effect of Vitamin D', *J Clin Endocrinol Metab*, **88** (2003), 10, 4623–32

18. Weiss, G. *et al.*, 'Immunomodulation by Perioperative Administration of n-3 Fatty Acids', *Br J Nutr*, **87** (2002), Supp 1, S89–94

19. Gissi-HF Investigators, 'Effect of n-3 Polyunsaturated Fatty Acids in Patients with Chronic Heart Failure (the GISSI-HF trial): A Randomised, Double-blind, Placebo-controlled Trial', *Lancet*, **372** (2008), 9645, 1223–30 and Gissi-HF Investigators, 'Effect of Rosuvastatin in Patients with Chronic Heart Failure (the GISSI-HF trial): A Randomised, Double-blind, Placebo-controlled Trial', *Lancet*, **372** (2008), 9645, 1231–9

20. Iso, H. *et al.*, 'Intake of Fish and Omega 3 Fatty Acids and Risk of Stroke in Women', *JAMA*, **285** (2001), 3, 304–12

21. Psota, T.L. *et al.*, 'Dietary Omega 3 Fatty Acid Intake and Cardiovascular Risk', *Am J Cardio*, **98** (2006), 4A, 3i–18i

22. Perez-Lopez, F.R., 'Vitamin D Metabolism and Cardiovascular Risk Factors in Post-menopausal Women', *Maturitas*, **62** (2009), 3, 248–62

23. Eliassen, A.H. *et al.*, 'Adult Weight Change and Risk of Postmenopausal Breast Cancer', *JAMA*, **296** (2006), 193–201

24. Palmieri, C. *et al.*, 'Serum 25-hydroxyvitamin D Levels in Early and Advanced Breast Cancer', *J Clin Pathol*, **59** (2006), 1334–6

25. Garland, C.F. *et al.*, 'The Role of Vitamin D in Cancer Prevention', *Am J Public Health*, **96** (2006), 252–61

26. Cho, E. *et al.*, 'Red Meat Intake and Risk of Breast Cancer among Premenopausal Women', *Arch Intern Med*, **166** (2006), 2253–9

27. Terry, P. *et al.*, 'Brassica Vegetables and Breast Cancer Risk', *JAMA*, **285** (2001), 23, 2975–7

28. Haggans, C.J. *et al.*, 'The Effect of Flaxseed and Wheat Bran Consumption on Urinary Oestrogen Metabolites in Premenopausal Women', *Cancer Epid Bio Prev*, **9** (2000), 719–725

29. Al Sarakbi, W. *et al.*, 'Dairy Products and Breast Cancer Risk: A Review of the Literature', *Int J Fertil Womens Med*, **50** (2005), 6, 244–9 and Alvarez-Leon, E.E. *et al.*, 'Dairy Products and Health: A Review of the Epidemiological Evidence', *Br J Nutr*, **96** (2006), Suppl, S94–9

30. Ganmaa, D. and Sato, A., 'The Possible Role of Female Sex Hormones in Milk from Pregnant Cows in the Development of Breast, Ovarian and Corpus Uteri Cancers', *Med Hypotheses*, **65** (2005), 1028–37

31. Ganmaa, D. and Sato, A., 'The Possible Role of Female Sex Hormones in Milk from Pregnant Cows in the Development of Breast, Ovarian and Corpus Uteri Cancers', *Med Hypotheses*, **65** (2005), 1028–37

32. Andrieu, N. *et al.*, 'Effect of Chest X-rays on the Risk of Breast Cancer among BRCA1/2 Mutation Carriers in the International BRCA1/2 Carrier Cohort Study: A Report from the EMBRACE, GENEPSO, GEO-HEBON, and IBCCS Collaborators' Group', *J Clin Oncol*, **24** (2006), 3361–6

33. Jorgensen, K.J. and Gotzsche, P.C., 'Who Evaluates Public Health Programmes? A Review of the NHS Breast Screening Programme', *J R Soc Med*, **103** (2010), 14–20

34. Gotzsche, P.C. and Nielsen, M., 'Screening for Breast Cancer with Mammography', *Cochrane Database Syst Rev*, **4** (2006), CD001877

35. Kaiser, L. *et al.*, 'Fish Consumption and Breast Cancer Risk: An Ecological Study', *Nutrition and Cancer*, **12** (1989), 61–8

36. Nkondjock, A. and Ghadirian, P., 'Intake of Specific Carotenoids and Essential Fatty Acids and Breast Cancer Risk in Montreal, Canada', *Am J Clin Nutr*, **79** (2004), 857–64

37. Shrubsole, M.J. *et al.*, 'Dietary Folate Intake and Breast Cancer Risk: Results from the Shanghai Breast Cancer Study', *Cancer Research*, **61** (2001), 7136–41

38. Lindau, S.T. and Gavrilova, 'Sex, Health and Years of Sexually Active Life Gained Due to Good Health: Evidence from Two US Population Based Cross Sectional Surveys of Ageing', *BMJ*, **340** (2010), 810

NOTES

39. Sangiovanni, J.P. *et al.*, 'Omega 3 Long Chain Polyunsaturated Fatty Acid Intake and 12 Year Incidence of Neovascular Age Related Macular Degeneration and Central Geographic Atrophy: A Prospective Cohort Study from the Age Related Eye Disease Study', *Am J Clin*, **90** (2009), 6, 1601–7

40. Age Related Eye Disease Study Research Group, 'A Randomised, Placebo Controlled, Clinical Trial of High Dose Supplementation with Vitamins C and E, Beta Carotene, and Zinc for Age Related Macular Denegation and Vision Loss', AREDS report No. 8, *Arch Opthalmol*, **119** (2001), 10, 417–36

41. Richer, S. *et al.*, 'Double Masked, Placebo Controlled, Randomised Trial of Lutein and Antioxidant Supplement in the Intervention of Atrophic Age Related Macular Degeneration: The Veterans LAST Study', Lutein Antioxidant Supplementation Trial, *Optometry*, **75** (2004), 4, 216–30

42. Bartlett, H. and Eperjesi, F., 'An Ideal Ocular Nutritional Supplement?', *Opthalimic Phsiol Opt*, **24** (2004), 4, 339–49

43. Gruenwald, J. *et al.*, 'Effect of Glucosamine Sulphate With or Without Omega 3 Fatty Acids in Patients with Osteoarthritis', *Adv Ther*, **26** (2009), 9, 858–71

44. Al Faraj, S. *et al.*, 'Vitamin D Deficiency and Chronic Low Back Pain in Saudi Arabia', *Spine*, **28** (2003), 2, 177–9

45. Ritchie, K. and Lovestone, S., 'The Dementias', *Lancet*, **360** (2002), 1759–66

46. Barberger-Gateau, P. *et al.*, 'Dietary Patterns and Risk of Dementia: The Three City Cohort Study', *Neurology*, **69** (2007), 20, 1921–30

47. Barberger-Gateau, P. *et al.*, 'Dietary Patterns and Risk of Dementia: The Three City Cohort Study', *Neurology*, **69** (2007), 20, 1921–30

48. Albanese, E. *et al.*, 'Dietary Fish and Meat Intake and Dementia in Latin America, China and India: A 10/6 Dementia Research Group Population Based Study', *Am J Clin Nutr*, **90** (2009), 2, 392–400

49. Chiu, C.C. *et al.*, 'The Effects of Omega 3 Fatty Acids Monotherapy in Alzheimer's Disease and Mild Cognitive Impairment: A Preliminary Randomised Double Blind Placebo Controlled Study', *Prog Neuropsychopharmacol Biol Psychiatry*, **32** (2008), 6, 1538–44

50. Yian Gu, *et al.*, 'Food Combination and Alzheimer Disease Risk: A Protective Diet', *Arch Neurol*, **67** (2010), 6

51. Barberger-Gateau, P. *et al.*, 'Dietary Patterns and Risk of Dementia: The Three City Cohort Study', *Neurology*, **69** (2007), 20, 1921–30

52. Zandi, P. *et al.*, 'Reduced Risk of Alzheimer's Disease in Users of Antioxidant Vitamin Supplements', *Arch Neurol*, **61** (2004), 82–8

53. Grundman, M., 'Vitamin E and Alzheimer's Disease: The Basis for Additional Clinical Trials', *Am J Clin Nutr*, **71** (2000), 630S–6S

54. Higgins, J.P. and Flicker, L., 'Lecithin for Dementia and Cognitive Impairment', *Cochrane Database Syst Rev*, **3** (2003) CD001015

55. Seshadri, S. *et al.*, 'Plasma Homocysteine as a Risk Factor for Dementia and Alzheimer's Disease', *NEJM*, **346** (2002), 476–83

56. Noble, J.M. *et al.*, 'Periodontitis is Associated with Cognitive Impairment among Older Adults: Analysis of NHANES-III', *J Neurol Neurosurg Psychiatry*, **80** (2009), 11, 1206–11

57. Rovio, S., *et al.*, 'Leisure Time Physical Activity at Midlife and the Risk of Dementia and Alzheimer's Disease', *Lancet Neurol*, **4** (2005), 11, 705–11

58. Friedland, R.P. *et al.*, 'Patients with Alzheimer's Disease have Reduced Activities in Midlife Compared with Healthy Control Group Members', *Proc Natl Acad Sci USA*, **98** (2001), 6, 3440–5

59. Suchy, J. *et al.*, 'Dietary Supplementation with a Combination of Alpha Lipoic Acid, Acetyl-L-carnitine, Glycerophosphocoline, Docosahexaenoic acid and Phosphatidylserine Reduces Oxidative Damage to Murine Brain and Improves Cognitive Performance', *Nutr Res*, **29** (2009), 1, 70–4

60. Weinmann, S. *et al.*, 'Effects of Ginkgo Biloba in Dementia: Systematic Review and Meta-analysis', *BMC Teriatr*, **10** (2010), 14

61. Martin, H.E. *et al.*, 'Interactions between Phytoestrogens and Human Sex Steroid Binding Protein', *Life Sci*, **58** (1996), 429–36

62. Haggans, C.J. *et al.*, 'Effect of Flaxseed Consumption on Urinary Estrogen Metabolites in Postmenopausal Women', *Nutr Canc*, **33** (1999), 188–95

INDEX

urethra 248, 266
urinary tract 8, 249
urine 43, 39, 45, 128, 182, 195, 213, 265
Utrogestan 186, 188

vagina 8, 12, 14, 135, 248, 249, 250,
    252, 266, 267
vaginal
  birth 266
  dryness 10, 116, 131, 250, 252
    and itching 247–49
  lubrication 16, 118, 122, 249, 252
vegetables 31–33, 158, 241
  cruciferous 47, 89, 106, 173, 261
vitamin A 32, 75, 86, 127, 171, 204,
    264
vitamin B 161, 214
vitamin B1 123
vitamin B2 123, 154
vitamin B3 154
vitamin B5 154
vitamin B6 30, 31, 58, 60, 87, 105, 154,
    233, 262
  pyridoxal-5 phosphate 58, 59, 60, 132
  pyridoxine hydrochloride 58, 59
vitamin B12 54, 87, 123, 205, 233, 262
vitamin C 32, 55, 59, 75, 78, 84, 86,
    128, 139, 156, 161, 169, 174,
    200, 204, 206, 248–49, 252, 254,
    261, 267, 268, 270
  Vitamin C Plus 129
vitamin D 54, 57, 80, 127, 171, 173,
    214, 216, 217, 221, 222, 223,
    228, 233, 236–37, 240, 256
  and breast health 240
  and inflammation 80
  and prevention of cancer 274
  and the ageing process 80
  blood tests 117, 273, 274
  deficiency 80–81, 247
  D2 (ergocalciferol) 59
  D3 (cholecalciferol) 59, 205
vitamin E 32, 75, 84–85, 86, 127, 174,
    204, 252, 261, 264
  d-alpha-tocopherol 59, 85
vitamin K 201, 215–16
  K1 215
  K2 215, 216, 223

vitamins
  B vitamins 45, 46, 56, 87, 123, 127,
    134, 154–55, 171, 205, 233, 264,
    271
    and stress 205
vomiting 122, 179, 218

warfarin 216
water 38–39, 89, 106, 203, 268
  drinking sufficient 159, 265
  loss 151
  retention 119, 129, 238
weight 5, 7, 28, 202
  being overweight 104, 145, 148–57,
    226, 227
  being underweight 147, 170–73, 258
  gain 10, 19, 32, 42, 48, 129, 131,
    147, 148, 162, 178, 251, 257–58
  how to control 147–74
  loss 40, 87, 145, 155, 141, 152, 160,
    161, 164, 167, 168, 170, 171, 172,
    178, 226, 258
    exercise and 143–45
    low-fat diets and 150
    my 10 golden rules for 157–61
    sleep and 92–93, 157
    the nine weight loss mistakes a
      woman can make 153
    too quick 158
  low body 116
  management 36, 38, 161, 257–58
  training 68, 143–45, 153, 158, 159,
    208, 258
womb (uterus) 14, 22, 23, 131, 135,
    136
  endometrial hyperplasia 121
  endometriosis 11, 104
  endometrium 14, 185, 186, 190

xenoestrogens 23, 35, 46, 103–6, 110,
    119, 242, 243

'Yes' 249
yoga 144–45, 146, 168, 208, 238

zeaxanthin 88
zinc 133, 155–56, 166, 223